YOGA FOR ATHEISTS RATIONALISTS
LOGICAL THINKERS AND NON-BELIEVERS

A DIY GUIDE

RAKESH SAINI

A Complete Do-it-yourself Guide For
Full Transformation and Betterment of Life Through Yoga

Following Stepwise Procedure of

45 * 45 (Learn 45 minutes daily for 45 days)
45 * 145 (Practise 45 minutes daily for 145 days)

for

Atheists, Rationalists, Logical Thinkers, and Non-Believers

rakeshsaini27@yahoo.com
rakeshsainirathore@gmail.com
@rakeshsaini27
rakeshsainiblog.wordpress.com
+91 9598901510, + 91 8174033723

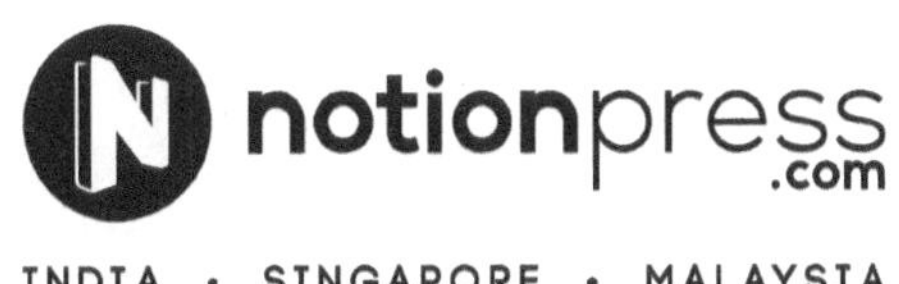

INDIA • SINGAPORE • MALAYSIA

Notion Press

Old No. 38, New No. 6
McNichols Road, Chetpet
Chennai - 600 031

First Published by Notion Press 2019
Copyright © Rakesh Saini 2019
All Rights Reserved.

ISBN 978-1-64587-084-5

Disclaimer

This guidebook is aimed at breaking the barriers and dispelling the negative myths about Yoga, existing in the minds of the atheists, rationalists, logical thinkers, non-believers and the ones with strong scientific tempers.

This book is also about increasing the knowledge and awareness about the importance of Meditation (Dhyana) (ध्यान), the Breathing exercises (Pranayama) (प्राणायाम), the Subtle Physical exercises (ShukshmaVyayam) (सूक्ष्मव्यायाम) and Yoga Asanas (The Physical postures) (योगासन) for enhancing one's physical, mental and existential wellbeing. The information given here is aimed at helping you make informed choices about your wellbeing, in totality.

It is not intended to serve any purpose connected with cure of ailments and diseases. This guide book is not at all connected with any healing sciences. It is not aimed at providing a substitute for any medical procedure or treatment.

Some of the Asanas/Exercises described here may require utmost care and abundant precautions. Else, they may harm the individual, particularly, if not performed properly, or the person is not completely fit.

If you are suffering from any medical conditions, you must consult doctors or experts before attempting any of the exercises. One must completely understand the precautions and benefits, pros and cons of the exercises described, before attempting any of the exercises.

Contents

Preface   *11*

How to Use This Guide   *17*

Acknowledgements   *25*

Chapter-One

Introduction, Basics, Precautions, Preparations and Postures

Day-One: Introduction   29
The Myths, Magic and Mystic of Yoga

Day-Two: Basics of Yoga: Part – I   36
Before We Begin

Day-Three: Basics of Yoga: Part – II   44
Before We begin

Day-Four: Basics of Yoga: Part – III   52
Learn before You Leap

Day-Five: Basics of Yoga: Part – IV   67
Preliminary Precautions

Day-Six: The Yogic Postures: Part – I   72
Basics and Hands Formations (HASTA-MUDRA)

Day-Seven: The Yogic Postures: Part – II   84
Yogic Postures for Relaxation

Day-Eight: The Yogic Postures: Part – III   93
                  Yogic Postures Suitable for Meditation
                  and Pranayama

Day-Nine: The Yogic Postures: Part – IV   101
                  The Starting Postures (Base Positions)

Day-Ten: Your Weekend Detoxification (Detox) Package   110

Chapter-Two

Meditation

Day-Eleven: Chanting for Fun and Relaxation   117

Day-Twelve: Ohm ('AUM') Chanting and Recitations 121

Day-Thirteen: Mantra Chanting   130

Day-Fourteen: Say Your Prayers   134

Day-Fifteen: Basics of Meditation Practices   142

Chapter-Three

Pranayama

Day-Sixteen: Breathing for Fun   149

Day-Seventeen: Basics of Pranayama   159

Day-Eighteen: Easy, Effective, Everyday Pranayama: Part – I   166

Day-Nineteen: Easy, Effective, Everyday Pranayama: Part – II   174

Day-Twenty: Some More Pranayama Exercises   179

Day Twenty-One: Packaged Stress Busters: Part – I   185

Day Twenty-Two: Packaged Stress Busters: Part – II   198

Day Twenty-Three: Create Your Own Package of Meditation
                    and Pranayama   204
                    Your Own Patented Stress Buster

Chapter-Four

The Subtle Exercises (Yogic Sukshma-Vyayama)

Day Twenty-Four: Yogic Sukshma–Vyayama
                    (The Subtle Exercises)   211

Day Twenty-Five: The Subtle Exercises for
                    Spinal System: Part – I   215

Day Twenty-Six: The Subtle Exercises for
                    Spinal System: Part – II   223

Day Twenty-Seven: The Subtle Exercises for Legs: Part – I   228

Day Twenty-Eight: The Subtle Exercises for Legs: Part – II 234

Day Twenty-Nine: The Subtle Exercises for Hands: Part – I 245

Day-Thirty: The Subtle Exercises for Hands: Part – II 251

Day Thirty-One: The Subtle Exercises for Neck   256

Day Thirty-Two: The Subtle Exercises in Lying
                    down Postures: Part – I   260

Day Thirty-Three: The Subtle Exercises in
                    Lying down Postures: Part – II   265

Day Thirty-Four: The Subtle Exercises for Upper Body and
                    Cardiac System   278

Day Thirty-Five: The Subtle Exercises in Standing Postures 285

Day Thirty-Six: The Subtle Exercises for Eyes 293

Day Thirty-Seven: Make Your Own Package of Subtle Exercises 301

Chapter-Five

The Yogic Postures (Yoga Asanas)

Day Thirty-Eight: The Yoga Asana in Standing Posture: Part – I 311

Day Thirty-Nine: The Yoga Asana in Standing Postures: Part – II 320

Day Forty: The Yoga Asana in Sitting Postures 325

Day Forty-One: The Yoga Asana in Lying down Posture 332

Day Forty-Two: Ending Your Daily Yoga Session 339

Day Forty-Three: Create Your Own Package for Daily Practice 349

Day Forty-Four: The Yogic Way of Life 352

Day Forty-Five: Concluding Remarks 360

Preface

This book is not about 'Dhyan' (Meditation), 'Pranayama' (the breathing exercises), 'Sukshma-Vyayama' (the subtle physical exercises) and 'Yoga' (the 'Asanas'). There are thousands of books on each of these subjects. There are many guide books available on Yoga. There are also millions of teachers for teaching the subjects.

If you have purchased this book, believing this to be a text book on Yoga, I request you to immediately return this book to the retailer and claim refund. Also, if you are reading this book to master the art and science of Yoga, I request you to stop immediately and not waste your time and energy. There are many books better than this. There are also many teachers better than me. I shall also be deliberately avoiding efforts towards defining Yoga, educating you on its history and delving into the intricate theories and benefits of Yoga, given in ancient texts.

This book is for those who have lots of misconceptions about Yoga. This book is aimed at dispelling many myths, pre-conceived notions, misinterpretations and misconceptions associated with Yoga.

This book is for atheists, who reject the concept of God, and therefore refuse to believe anything that is associated with God.

This guide is for those believing Yoga to be a proprietary article of Hindus and their gods. I am a firm atheist. I believe that the marketers and teachers have, so far not done full justice to this subject. Yoga is a universal Art and Science of wellbeing, and for happy, healthy and peaceful living. By associating the subject with ancient Hindu texts, predominantly Hindu

Sages and Saints, they have closed the doors for those who hate either the religion or the Hindus, for whatsoever reasons.

This book is for rational and logical thinkers, who believe in mostly westernised concepts of modern science and vehemently refuse to accept anything associated with ancient arts and sciences.

This book is for those who are obsessed with their own reasons in disliking religions originating from the Indian continent; those who believe Hindus to be saffron-clad monks, snake-charmers, tribals or peasants; those who look at Buddhists only as spirituality-obsessed, pot-bellied, laughing Buddhas. A Sikh for them is a warrior, ready to wield the kirpan at the slightest provocation. They may look at Jainism as nothing more than vegetarianism. This guide is aimed at leading them on a path to Yoga, circumventing all the trappings of religion and spirituality.

This book is for those who hate the concept of religion. I also firmly believe that religion, as a concept, deserves to be hated. Over the years religion has done more harm to humanity and human civilisation, than good. Most religions divide, preach hatred for other religions, promote superstitions and in extreme cases promote violence.

Yoga, on the other hand derives its name itself form unity. Yoga is all about unification and addition. Unification of one with his inner-self, nature, environment, surroundings, family, health, mental peace, and society is Yoga. Yoga is all about positivity. The only subtraction relevant to Yoga is with bodily diseases, mental-unrest, and emotional-instability, i.e., all negatives. The modern sciences and management principles are nowhere in conflict with Yoga.

This book is also for those believing that popping too many pills, when fallen ill, is the best method to keep oneself healthy. The modern medical sciences, particularly Allopathic Sciences, driven by greed of the megabucks pharmaceutical industry, leave no stone unturned in propagating the myth that pills are the best cure and all other formats of healthy living or medical treatments are nothing but quackery. Popping too many pills is harmful for health, wellbeing and wealth. Yoga, if nothing else, at least teaches you a system of remaining healthy, without popping too many pills.

This book is of immense relevance for Muslims, Christians and those professing religions and the ways of living other than 'Hinduism.' Particularly, those who have been taught by their religious preachers and teachers, that all religions, other than their own, are either inferior to, or in conflict with their religion.

Yoga teaches us the ways and means of remaining happy and healthy. All other methods of keeping oneself physically fit, mentally agile, defying age, attaining inner peace and contentment may also be good. If you are the one practising any Art or Science of such nature, do try Yoga also. You are likely to discover yourself that Yoga is superior to your methods.

You may also end up picking some elements of your practices and adding those to Yogic methods and creating a new improved method of physical and mental fitness. If you believe in experimenting with your body, mind, heart and soul, I humbly request you to try Yoga. You may also be tempted to pen down a book on new methods developed by you, by experimentation, just as the writer himself.

This book is also for those who have in the past attempted learning Yoga through books, videos or teachers and have given up, due to disinterest, lack of learning, failure to translate into daily and routine practices, intimidation due to complexity of Asanas and practices or any other reasons. Please try it once again, by following the principles that I am trying to teach in this book. You are at zero risk. I am one amongst you. I also failed many times.

I earn my bread and butter by working in an environment surrounded by men from Army, Navy, and Air Force. All fighting fit. The envy, the jealousy and the desire to not feel inferior to them, in physical fitness standards, propelled me to search for a package of practices to remain healthy, without going into the extremes of Military Drills. This led me to experimenting with a few formats of exercises. Yoga, amongst them, was least acceptable and palatable to my taste. However, after failing with others, I kept on trying and experimenting with Yoga. Finally, not only did I succeed but I got trapped to the extent that I feel I should now help others, similarly placed.

This book is more about the results of my experimentation and observations on my body, heart and mind, than acquisition of theoretical knowledge form books and teachers. This statement should in no way take away credits form the authors of books that I have read and teachers who taught me. I acknowledge the contributions of some of the great books and teachers, who have greatly influenced not only this book, but my entire lifestyle, wellbeing and thought process. To name one or a few will be injustice to many remaining unnamed.

Yoga cures many physical ailments. However, this book does not claim to be a treatise on curing ailments. If you are suffering from any disease and looking for an alternative treatment, do try Yoga. I advise you to pick up some other good book, after your initiation into Yoga following my methods, on treatment methodology of Yoga and Ayurveda or read books relevant to the illness. Do not depend on this book for treatment. In any case, do consult your medical practitioner before attempting any of the Asanas.

If you are a beginner, trying to learn the art and science of Yoga, this is the right place for you. I have attempted to make the learning process simple and effective. You may find many new and interesting things here, which a proper and trained Yoga teacher will never tell you. You will also not find many concepts and learnings described here, in any other book. They are not to be blamed. They have learnt their skills from some School or Institute of Yoga.

Each School, Institute, Camp, Teacher believes in a specific way of Yogic Science. They are also keen to retain the purity and sanctity of their form of Yoga. I may, in fact be blamed for polluting and reducing to pulp, the pure, sanguine and divine sense of Yoga. However, my aim is to make Yoga accessible to those who have closed their door to it. Once you enter and find it interesting and beneficial, do read other advanced books, or go to a trained teacher.

You might have seen some complicated, intimidating Yogic practices, in the past. Those involving twisting and turning of body parts, as if there are no bones in the body, defying gravity and turning the belly area better than a trained belly dancer. Or if you are carrying images of Yogis standing on head, on toes, or on one foot for days together and you felt fear and intimidation, this is the right place for you. Yoga is not those practices alone. Those practices are a minor part of Yoga.

Those practices are for those who, having mastered their craft, want themselves to be elevated to some other level. You and I do not fall into that bracket. We are common men. We are leading our life the normal way. We want our practice to give us peace, good health and happiness. We want Yoga to aid and abet our normal living. We want Yoga to complement our life and not complicate it. I have avoided all such advanced and complicated practices in this guide.

If you are the ones who firmly believe that money is everything in life, that money can buy you all health, happiness and peace, this guide is useless for you. This will cause you no harm and no good.

If you believe that peace is supreme, happiness is precious, and health is non-negotiable, non-sellable and not available in malls and markets, my hopes and aspirations are hinged on you. I expect, I aspire, and I hope to earn a Thank You Note/a Card/a Mail or some silent applause/appreciation/ thanks from you, for all my troubles, midnight-LEDs burnings, trials and hard work of more than six months, after your adoption of Yoga in life and six to seven months of routine practices.

You may also look at my effort here, as that of sieving and filtering Yoga. Making the palatable and consumable essential ingredients of Yoga separate from difficult to decipher concepts of spirituality, unification with God, intricate religious packaging and superstitious looking elements. I am serving you here a perfectly sieved and filtered part of Yoga.

I once again acknowledge the great Sages and Saints, the great teachers, experimenters, authors, writers, video-creators and all other contributors to the great Art and Science of Yoga. They have created a huge body of work, of immense value for the benefit of humanity. We just need to pick a few ounces from this great heap to keep ourselves happy, healthy, content, satisfied and peaceful and to excel in life. If you like this book, do tell others. If you hate it, I shall be waiting for your brickbats, with a wide grin on my face and a big thank you.

Are you ready for it?
Do I hear yes?
All right, then let's start learning!
Respectful Regards
Rakesh Saini

rakeshsaini27@yahoo.com
rakeshsainirathore@gmail.com
@rakeshsaini27
rakeshsainiblog.wordpress.com

How to Use This Guide

I strongly recommend, that in the first instance, you read this book like any other fiction, non-fiction, self-improvement and Do-It-Yourself (DIY) guides.

Thereafter, decide if you want to imbibe Yoga in your life. Please note that I am not asking you to decide 'if you want to learn Yoga.' Learning is no big deal. You have millions of options. But Yoga is not a set of exercises to be learnt, practised and repeated daily. It is a way of life. You must change your lifestyle. You must implant Yoga in your life and imbibe Yogic practices in your daily routines. There are no short-cuts. There is no place for half-learners.

I am not saying that you must transform yourself into monks, quit smoking, quit drinking and lead a sedentary life. Contrary to popular perceptions, I believe that Yoga helps you in enjoying all these ills, ills as perceived by society at large.

But, there are certain changes that you must make. They will all add and enhance your personality, your stature and your aura.

The first and foremost change is commitment of devoting at least forty-five minutes of your valuable time, preferably early in the morning to yourself.

The second commitment you must make to yourself and me is to devote forty-five days for learning. I have carefully crafted here a sequential learning process, requiring minimum forty-five days.

The third condition is that you have faith in me. First, believe in everything that I say. Follow the routines, the instructions blindly. Once you attain some proficiency, do feel free to conduct your own research or experimentation and prove me wrong.

Lastly, do not stop practising and do not stop learning. You must practise your own routines, which you will create during learning for at least 145 days after completing learnings. Yoga requires at least that much of time to show results and improvements. No matter whatsoever proficiency level you reach, you will always find new and better things to learn in Yoga.

Interested? Despite my forewarnings? I am repeating. Yoga is addictive. Once you start enjoying the fruits of good health, happy mood, may be more respect or promotion at work, you won't be able to go back. It is a vicious circle. I got stuck into this like a fly in a spider's web. Now, I want you here for company. Do not blame me later.

Having made your decision, I request you to devote forty-five minutes every day early morning for practising, experimenting, learning and perfecting the forty-five sets of exercise-packages I present here. Be punctual. Be a disciplined, obedient learner. Remember 'Yama' and 'Niyama' being important organs of Yoga.

Create Your Resume

At the very outset, may I request you for a favour? Now that you have invested money in purchasing this book, I do not think you have very many options. You may as well concede to my request and grant me the favour. This exercise will prove to be beneficial to both of us, you and me.

I want you to create your own resume, your own self-assessment. It is not the professional kind of resume needed for job applications. It is a physical, lifestyle and emotional kind of self-assessment. You need to reflect on at least the last six months of your past life and build up an honest, candid self-assessment for your own personal use. There are no identity-theft issues involved here. It is your bio data, created by you, with you and for your benefit only. So democratic! Let me guide you in building up this self-assessment.

Take Some Photographs

Resume is not complete without a photograph. I am not asking for a passport or stamp size photograph, but a portfolio of photographs. You may conveniently click a few selfies on your Smartphone. This portfolio should include a few close-ups of your face, a few normally standing full postures from two or three angles, and a few photos of normally sitting postures on chair, desk or work-station.

Physical Attributes

Next contents of your resume should be your physical attributes. It should contain your height, weight, Body Mass Index (BMI), blood pressure, blood sugar levels, heart beat rate, breathing speed (inhalations per minute), your heart conditions, lungs conditions, kidney functioning, eye sights, medical history (last six months), records of diseases or infections (minor/major) suffered, your food habits, your exercise routines including time spent per day/week, your work routines and your overall lifestyle and persona.

Emotional Attributes

This may be somewhat difficult to understand. You may also find it difficult to remain honest and loyal to yourself. I request you to diligently and sincerely assess your emotional attributes, your emotional quotient, for both positive and negative emotions.

How many times do you openly, heartily, unashamedly laugh in a day? How many times does a wide smile appear on your face, how many times is an urge, hunger and pang of creativity felt? You feel like picking a brush for painting a beautiful painting, or a thought comes to your mind bringing a yearning for penning down a poem or a piece of prose, or you wish to create a sculpture, or you wish to pick up a new hobby, a new learning, or simply want to sing a melodious beautiful song. These are very strong indicators of positive emotions.

Similarly, include the set of negative emotions of stress, anger, irritation, fear, jealousy, depression, etc. To quantify, you may assess how many times you feel irritation over a small issue, you are angry, you feel depressed, you are fearful of some bad news coming your way, you lose your temper, you shout at your subordinates, colleagues or family members, etc., etc.

You may write down all these in a descriptive manner, in paragraphs of say 2500–3000 words or you may write down the above questions and award yourself a score from 1 to 10, using your own criteria of scoring.

You can thus create a matrix of your physical attributes and positive and negative emotions. Call it your physical-emotional matrices. Only after your Paragraph/Matrix is ready, continue further readings. Keep this to yourself, you may store it in your laptop/Tab/Smartphone or preserve the paper carefully. I will at the end of this book tell you what to do with this, in my 'concluding remarks.'

Okay!… Guys and Girls!… Ladies and Gentlemen….! are you now ready to traverse this path with me? Are you ready to be my companion on this highway named **"45 * 45 and 45 * 145"** (Forty-five minutes of learning/practising per day, forty-five days of learning and 145 days of practising routinely for forty-five minutes per day after learning).

Do I hear yes?
Can you loudly scream Yeeeeessssssssss!
Let the learning begin!

This DIY guide is organised in five chapters. Each Chapter is divided into five to fourteen Sections, named as Days to correspond with the expected time that you should take to read, assimilate and do some preliminary practices of that section.

Chapter-One, titled 'Introduction, Basics, Precautions, Preparations and Postures' comprising of ten days, is your introductory drill.

I firmly believe that the epicentre of our reluctance in adoption of Yoga lies in those two loafs of blood-stained flesh, encased within our skull, commonly known as 'brain' or 'mind.' Taming and regulating the mind are the most important prerequisites to facilitate its adoption.

The mind is also a major contributor of negativities in your life. Acknowledging this primacy of the brain, the Yogic prescription of 'meditation' as the tricks and techniques to tame and regulate the brain, is part of your learnings in Chapter-Two.

Chapter-Three consisting of eight days is devoted to 'Pranayama,' the art of regulating breath.

'Sukshma-Vyayama' is one of the most important parts of physical exercise in Yoga. In Chapter-Four comprising of fourteen sections (days) you will learn these subtle physical exercises.

The subject matter of Chapter-Five is the most visible and popular part of Yoga 'the Yoga Asana.' It is divided into nine sections/days.

For each day some new lessons are included and named as 'Learning for the day.' Each section may also invariably contain some sub-sections as, 'Practice for the day,' 'Tutorial for the day,' 'Tip of the day' and 'Table of the day.'

You are expected to read the Sub-Section 'Learning for the day' in the first fifteen to twenty minutes of the forty-five minutes that you have allocated to yourself and committed to me. If a Sub-Section "Practice for the day" is included, please devote the rest of the time to practice and master the asana/exercise/practice taught.

Tutorials are your homework. Some activities in the nature of exploration are given as tutorials. Tips are of course tips. The tables are summaries and are to serve the purpose of easy reference and ease of recollection.

Some practices may require some specific precautions. All precautions are given at the beginning. Observe those precautions diligently. Also, some practices are initially considered difficult. Such practices are indicated as difficult in the very beginning. Do exercise due care in attempting these exercises.

Some sub-sections are marked as 'For academic interest only.' These are merely included for the sake of knowing and awareness. They do not play a significant role in your learning, practising and adopting Yoga.

My pledges and my promises are as follows. Kindly recollect and re-pledge your commitments.

My pledge:

You give me:

- **Forty-five minutes of your valuable time for forty-five days to learn.**
- **Forty-five minutes of your valuable time every day for 145 days for practice.**

I return back:

- **A refreshed, rejuvenated, revitalised, detoxed, healthy and happy you.**

With:

- **A package of practices.**
- **To serve you for lifetime.**
- **To reduce your medical and insurance costs.**
- **A support system to fall back upon when in stress, distress or disease.**

Without:

- Changing your religion.
- Changing your belief system.
- Changing your thought process about origin of life and God.
- Turning you into a saffron-clad Sadhu, Monk, Yogi or 'Bhramachari.'

My Promise:

- To make your learning smooth, and enjoyable.
- To make scientific explanations as simple as feasible.
- To not use complex, heavy, Hindi and Sanskrit words and phrases.

Are you game for it?

Yes!

Let's play then!

Acknowledgements

I acknowledge the contributions of all Indian Saints, Sages, Yogis and the learned, enlightened souls, who conceived the mesmerizingly beautiful art and science of Yoga, in ancient times.

I acknowledge the contributions of Saint Patanjali, who assembled and assimilated this package of practices, and perhaps gave it an apt name, Yoga, to signify addition and unification. A name, so appropriate and so beautiful, that one can derive thousands of meanings and millions of interpretations.

I also acknowledge the contributions of the modern-day Yogis, Gurus and Teachers. They have made yeoman contributions in popularising, propagating, and making the masses aware of this beautiful art and science. Particularly the contributions of Late Shi B K S Iyengar, Baba Ramdev of Patanjali Yogapeeth, Shri Shri Ravi Shankar of Art of Living, and Shri Jaggi Vasudev of Isha Foundation are respectfully recognised. Their immense body of work has inspired millions.

I acknowledge the contributions of Shri Narendra Modi, Honourable Prime Minister of India, whose untiring efforts culminated in the United Nations General Assembly (UNGA), unanimously declaring 21 June as "International Day of Yoga" also called as "Yoga Day." His efforts not only resulted in Yoga gaining global acceptance and universal awareness, but also enhanced its acceptance and sense of pride in India.

I also acknowledge the efforts of Researchers and Scientists, mostly in Western Countries, who revived and resuscitated this science, after its deliberate belittling and destruction during Mughal and British rules in India.

I also express my gratitude to Late Dr. K.M. Ganguli, of Dr. Ganguli Yoga Vidhyapeeth, Bhopal, Madhya Pradesh, (India) and his dedicated, devoted team of disciples, who are making sustained efforts to keep up the good work started by Dr. Ganguli.

I am also inspired by the books of Dr. Shamsher Prakash (an eminent Professor of Civil Engineering, at University of Roorkee, India, and an equally renowned Yoga-Acharaya) of Shamsher Prakash Foundation, Swami Satyananda Saraswati and other eminent teachers of Bihar School of Yoga. Their teaching contained in various books have been personally adopted, practised and incorporated in this guide, in one or the other way. I also express my gratitude towards my Parents.

Chapter-One

Introduction, Basics, Precautions, Preparations and Postures

Chapter–One

Day-One: Introduction

The Myths, Magic and Mystic of Yoga

Learning for the Day

Yoga derives its name from terms which describe binding, joining, attaching, adding, combining and yoking. It is an evolved science. Evolved out of observations of nature, animal life and plant life, by learned, enlightened men in ancient times. The science is evolved out of experimentation by saints and seers in quest of physical wellbeing, mental peace, contentment, enlightenment and attainment of inner peace.

The Honourable Prime Minister of India, Shri Narendra Modi, while delivering his address at the 69th session of the UNGA on September 27, 2014, described Yoga as:-

"Yoga is an invaluable gift of ancient Indian tradition. It embodies unity of mind and body, thoughts and action, restraint and fulfilment, harmony between men and nature and a holistic approach to health and wellbeing. Yoga is not about exercise, but to discover the sense of oneness with ourselves, the World and Nature. By changing our lifestyle and creating consciousness, it can help us to deal with climate change. Let us work towards adopting an International Yoga day."

This to my mind, sums up all that modern-day Yoga is. It is an art of controlling your mind, the supercomputer, encased in your skull. It is an art of channelizing your mental energy and guiding it to flow, the way you desire.

It is an art of acquiring command over your emotions. An art aimed at enhancing all your positive emotions of love, respect, regard, compassion, contentment, peace, happiness, satisfaction, gratefulness, deriving pleasure in wellbeing and happiness of others, and betterment of nature, environment and the universe. It is an art of keeping on a tight leash all your negative emotions of envy, ego, jealousy, greed, and violence.

Yoga is the science of keeping your complete body, i.e., the skeleton, spine, bones, muscles, nerves, senses, sensors and receptors, transmitters, control systems, regulators and the communication systems, all healthy and fit.

"Yoga is not an ancient myth buried in oblivion. It is the most valuable inheritance of the present. It is the essential need of today and the culture of tomorrow."

– Swami Satyananda Saraswati

Yoga traces its origin to the Indian continent. So do many religions, Hinduism, Buddhism, Jainism and Sikhism being the prominent ones. The evolution of Yoga and these religions was concurrent. Therefore, there is a marked similarity in the preaching and practices of Yoga and these religions. This is expected. In those times the human mind was also not so evolved. The capabilities of the human mind were also developing, breaking out of their shackles.

Therefore, it was easier for the learned and enlightened ones amongst the general masses, to preach both at the same time and place. This seems to be the only reason for the Indian religious concepts intermingling with Yogic concepts.

Yoga otherwise is a universal art and a universal science. The unanimous adoption of an International Day of Yoga (Yoga day) by UNGA is a proof, if one was ever needed.

The ancient texts describe eight limbs or stages of Yoga *('Ashtanga-Yoga')* as under: *(For academic interest only):-*

Yama: (Adherence to, respect for universal moral commandants, respect for universal laws of Nature)—Controls the passions and emotions and keeps one in harmony with his fellow men, the nature and the universe. Non-violence *('Ahimsa')*, Truth *('Satya')*, Non-stealing *('Asteya')*, Self-control *('Brahmacharya')* and Un-selfishness *('Aparigraha')* are believed to be five important *'Yamas.'*

Niyama: (Adherence to Rule of Law, Self-discipline, self-purification by discipline)—also controls the passions and emotions and keeps a person in harmony with his fellow men, the nature and the universe. Cleanliness *('Saucha')*, Contentment *('Santosha')*, Sustained efforts *('Tapas')*, Self-study *('Svadhyaya')* and faith in creator *('Ishvar-Pranidhana')* are important *'Niyamas.'*

Asana: (The postures)—Keeps the body healthy, fit, strong and in harmony with the environment.

Pranayama: (The controlled, rhythmic breathing—inhalation, exhalation and retention)

Pratyahara: (Control of mind, withdrawal and emancipation of mind from the dominance of the senses and exterior objects)

Dharana: (The concentration, the focus)

Dhyana: (The meditation)

Samadhi: (A state of super-consciousness, an extreme elevated enlightenment, reached by the practitioner by sustained and profound meditation, in which the practitioner unites with, and become one with the object of his meditation, i.e., the Creator)

There are many different traditional schools, each with its own unique philosophy, traditions, teaching methodology and package of practices. Some of these are; *JNANA YOGA, BHAKTI YOGA, KARMA YOGA, PATANJALI YOGA, KUNDALINI YOGA, HATHA YOGA, DHAYANA YOGA, MANTRA YOGA, LAYA YOGA, RAJA YOGA, JAIN YOGA, BOUDDHA YOGA,* etc.

In recent times, it has become a fashion to assign a hip, modern, fashionable, designer, stylish terminology with Yoga. Some such terms are; *KRIYA YOGA, TANTRA YOGA, SIDH YOGA, TRANSCENDENTAL MEDITATION YOGA, TIBETAN YOGA, VIPASANA, HOT YOGA, SUDARSHAN KRIYA YOGA, CHRISTIAN YOGA, MINDFUL YOGA, BEER YOGA, NUDE YOGA, NAKED YOGA, etc.* Sometimes, a particular branch of Yoga claims to get magical results.

Please understand that, if you get your basics right, you need not bother about these fancy names. You may even devise a new name, a new school yourself, say *IT – YOGA, DIGITAL – YOGA, Smartphone – YOGA, i-YOGA, e-YOGA or SELFI –YOGA* and market it. So, pay adequate attention and get the basics right!

According to ancient text books on Yoga:- *(For academic interest only. I have no scientific proofs/explanations)*

- There are 84,00,000 Yoga postures *('Asanas').* The numbers of incarnations that one must mandatorily pass through before attaining liberation *('Moksha'),* from the painful cycle of births and deaths, were also believed to be 84,00,000 in ancient Hindu texts. So, there was originally one Yogic posture for each stage of liberation. Look, how thoughtful, balanced and harmonious our ancestors were! Do not get intimidated by these numbers. You are not required to learn this vast set. Even if you just master 84, you are an acknowledged beginner, master two times (168 Asanas) and you become an accomplished practitioner. To earn your next promotion to 'Yoga Master'/Expert level, you perhaps just need to master 168 more Asanas.

- In 'Pranayama,' it is believed that during one's life cycle a person can have maximum 800 million breaths. Faster breathing shortens the life span and slower breathing enhances it. Present average breathing rate of a healthy person is sixteen per minute. If you can reduce your breathing rate to fifteen per minute, you may live up to hundred years. Mathematical extrapolation also reveals that if one can control the breathing rate to one in one minute, he can live up to 1500 years(?).

How Does Yoga Work?

Yoga is unity of two existing substances. It is essentially the full concentration of the mind over the body parts, exercised in Yogic postures. Comfortable positioning of body in some specific postures and holding it, with joy, concentration of mind and senses and awareness of breath are Yogic postures.

Your body is made up of millions and millions of cells and a framed mobile structure. They need constant nourishment, maintenance and repair. The mobility demands lubrication. Yoga not only nourishes the tissues and cells but also tones up the whole bodily systems and helps proper blood circulation and proper removal of waste products and residues. Regular practice of Yoga keeps joints and spine supple, strong and flexible.

In the modern day, given the corporate, industrial, competitive ways of working and distorted lifestyles and life-patterns, sparing time for oneself has become a big challenge. Yoga offers the methods by which one can remain fit by spending fifteen to ninety minutes daily, as per availability of time.

While other formats of physical exercises work largely on the physical levels (bones and muscles), Yoga works on the internal organs of our body on seven systems that run parallel, concurrently and complimentarily. These are:

- Nervous System

- Respiratory System

- Circulatory System

- Digestive System

- Absorption System

- Excretory System

- Reproductive System

Yoga benefits the Endocrine System, which influences almost every cell, organ, and function of our bodies. The endocrine system is instrumental in regulating mood, growth and development, tissue functions, metabolism, sexual function and reproductive processes.

Yoga is an attitude, a discipline that transforms the way you live and conduct yourself. Yoga not only keeps you fit, disease-free, energetic and young but equips you with mental and physical strength and tenacity to face the ups and downs of life. Regular and sustained practice increases productivity at workplace, removes negativity from mind and toxins from the body, leading to sound sleep and tension-free life.

Even without my explanations and elaborations here, once you go through the forty-five days of learning, you will yourself appreciate that Yoga encompasses the finest of the following:

- Meditation

- Breathing exercises

- The subtle physical exercises, involving alternate stretching and relaxing of bones, muscles and nerves, in some specific manners

- The Yoga Asanas (postures designed to tone up, control, regulate or enhance and elevate the functioning of one or more of the organs, glands, muscles, nerves or control and regulatory systems)

- Bio-mimetic (Bio-mimicry) Science (concerning imitation of the models, systems, and elements of other forms of life (plants, animals) for solving complex human problems)

- Positive-auto-suggestions

- Alternative Healing and Medicinal Sciences: Ayur-Veda, (a traditional Indian healing science based on balances in bodily systems) Naturopathy, Acupuncture, Acupressure, Magnet therapy, Massage therapy, etc.

Yoga is apparently an easy form of exercising but is much more effective and beneficial in comparison to other traditional exercises. Yoga gives practitioners good health, stamina, higher working capacity and intelligence of mind. It also promotes adoption of one's zeal, enthusiasm towards life, clarity and purity of thoughts, leading one towards peace, happiness, joy, health and all-round development. This package, as a whole, is an 'absolute value for money (time)' and *full paisa-vasool.'*

You and I are actually very fortunate. We do not need to go to a *Panditji* (an astrologer) to find the auspicious time for *'Muhurat'* (Inauguration) of our learning. So what are we waiting for! Let the learning begin!

Day-Two: Basics of Yoga: Part – I
Before We Begin

I sincerely hope that you have respected my advice. You have, at least cursorily, gone through the contents of this guide from beginning to end, before coming back here again, with a commitment to spend forty-five minutes daily with me on this beautiful journey. If Yes! Let's start the journey! Bon Voyage to you! If Not! Kindly do not start any practice, until you acquire preliminary knowledge of the subject, in totality, by once reading this guide from beginning to end.

Learning for the Day

Before starting practising, it is important to understand a few basics and a few preliminary precautions.

Time

Time is of immense essence for all activities in everyday life. Time is of essence for life, work, family and society. Time is of immense essence for learning and practising Yoga too. Whereas you may decide to learn at any time of the day, (Look, how liberal I am! Giving you so much of freedom. Where else will you find such freedom?) the best time for learning, is early in the morning, before sunrise. The air is fresh and rich in oxygen. Your mind and body are also fresh after a good night's sleep.

The practising, however, must be done early in the morning on empty stomach, empty bowels and bladder, with clean mind and clean body. Only if despite best intentions you are unable to find time in the morning, you may practise in the evening. Ensure your belly is empty. Do not have any meal or snack, at least forty-five minutes before and after the practice session.

Empty Stomach, Clean Belly

The term 'empty stomach' needs to be clearly understood. It is a must that you have had your morning motions, but not sufficient. Your motions must result in an empty, clean and refreshed belly. If you are not much aware about the difference between having morning motions and a clean belly/ empty stomach, perform the test described as 'Test for empty stomach' under 'Tip of the day.' If you face difficulties in achieving the clean belly in the morning, try a few of the stunts described in Chapter – One, Day-Ten, 'Your Weekend Detox Package.'

Tip of the Day

Tip: Test for Empty Stomach
After exiting from washroom, press your belly inwards, utilising muscles in the stomach and without forced breathing and taxing your lungs. Hold the belly inward for a few seconds. Release automatically, without using too much energy of muscles or breath. Repeat five to ten times. Observe how you feel. Was it effortless? Was the upper skin of belly traversing enough to and fro distances? Was a cavity good enough to hold about ½ to 1 litre of water being formed? Was your belly skin feeling almost ready to touch the inner skin of your back? If the answer to all these queries is yes, congratulations! Your stomach is clean. Your belly is empty. You are ready to conquer the world.

Clean Body, Clean Mind

You should start your practice with clean body. It is preferable, though not mandatory, that you take a bath or shower before starting your session. If your body type is such that you sweat profusely during your sleep or climatic conditions are hot and humid, and you are not using air-conditioning (you deserve an award for taking care of the nature and the environment), you should better take a shower before your practise.

Place

Whereas you may choose any place, any posture, to enhance your learning by reading this book, the practice sessions must be performed at a neat and clean place. The best place is outdoors, in a garden or a park, with plenty of trees, bushes, shrubs and grass. The air surrounding you must be pure and with abundance of oxygen.

A few water bodies, lakes, fountains, waterfalls or some soothing sounds of flowing or falling water, and chirpings of birds, would be an icing on the cake. However, if you are unable to find such a place in your neighbourhood, you may practice indoors. The place however, must be neat, clean and airy with unobstructed flow of fresh outside air.

Do not use air-conditioning, even if you are addicted to it. Open the windows and let the fresh air get in and escape. For this, it is important to understand the natural wind-flow directions in your house. Identify and keep open two openings, perpendicular to the directions of natural flow of winds, opposite to each other. This will allow natural ventilation. If you haven't yet figured out the wind directions and their seasonal variations in your locality, it will be a fantastic idea to do some research without Googling and using your Smartphone. Move out one fine morning and find out, man! Trust me; it will be fun and enjoyable!

If the only place that you can find is indoors, centrally-heated or air-conditioned, make sure that your service provider takes adequate care of Indoor Air Quality (IAQ). You should also be familiar with the subject. If not, do some research and find out if the indoor air in your confined space meets the stipulated standards. While researching the subject of IAQ, you may also like to find out if you can improve it by some indoor plants. Do not normally use fans. If use of fan is unavoidable, it should rotate at slow speed, just enough to facilitate evaporation of mild sweat that you may get during intense practices.

Some added elements of a good fragrance, indoor fountain or waterfall, soothing colours, abundant greenery and some oxygen enriching potted plants shall enhance the benefits of your Yogic efforts.

Hydration

It is important that your body is adequately hydrated before you start any practice session. It is more important for smokers and casual social drinkers. It is not my present aim to dissuade you from these habits. You are aware, they are not good for your health. Regular practice sessions and imbibing Yogic way of living should help you in quitting such practices, provided you desire to do so and have the will to do so. For the time being, it is enough to understand that you will sweat out during your practices. Even if this sweating is not visible, your body will consume excess water during exercises. You should not experience any dehydration.

One should also not drink water or any other fluid at least ten to fifteen minutes before practice. It makes good sense to drink plenty of water, as first thing in the morning. Lukewarm water consumed early in the morning gives immense health benefits.

It is strongly recommended to drink at least one and a half litre of lukewarm water in the morning. Keep your electric kettle—or any other mode of heating water—buzzing. Drink as much water as feasible throughout the day. Do not bother about frequent urination. After all, for what purpose do you have a washroom at home and workplace? Keep your flush busy but do not waste too much of water. Just avoid drinking fluids ten to fifteen minutes before and after practice.

If you are a habitual consumer of your morning cuppa of tea or coffee and you are unable to start your morning routines without it, do continue doing so. Compensate your hydration by drinking two additional glasses of water for each cup of tea or coffee being consumed. Avoid excess sugar, cream and milk in tea/coffee.

Even if you do not see any apparent sign of sweating, do not assume that you are not sweating, or your body is not consuming excess water. Be very careful of your body-hydration.

Get Your Clothes Proper

You should be wearing minimal clothing during practice. Your clothes should be ventilating and absorbent. Fabric is very important. Your clothing's fabric should allow entry of fresh air down to the last pores of your body. It should absorb your sweat.

Thin cotton is best. You should wear loose clothing. Your clothes should allow smooth, musical and dance-like movements for all parts of your body. Some practices require rotation of your arms, legs, neck, etc. Clothes should not cause any obstruction in such movements. Wearing of tight undergarments should be avoided, if possible.

If you are practising outdoors, just wear as few clothes as are necessary to avoid public nudity. If indoors, wear as less as you are comfortable with in the presence of your family members, roommates or co-livers. Hey, remember, many of your family members, except your children, might have seen you naked at some time in the past. So, why bother too much about it.

(For guys) If comfortable, you may keep the upper part of your body open or wear a thin loose armless vest. Thin cotton boxer shorts are okay for the lower body. But please take care of that black hairy patch between your legs, if wearing whites. There is no point in making a public display of it. Please avoid the body hugging thick polyester clothes aggressively sold in the market as Yoga dresses.

(For girls) You are aware of how much your modesty permits you. Wear as much as that. But please avoid body hugging tight clothing. Clothes not allowing free passage of air and not absorbing water are a strict no-no.

I am not promoting nudity here. There is a specific branch, a school of Yoga called 'nude Yoga' or 'naked Yoga.' There is no harm in that. If you are home alone, not likely to be disturbed, by all means go ahead and try it. But this book is not about that branch or that school of Yoga.

Get Your Tools and Plants Proper

The beauty of Yoga is that unlike gym-ing, walking or many other formats of physical fitness requiring expensive tools and equipments, Yoga practice actually requires nothing. All that is required is a neat, clean surface covering that may provide your full body, when fully stretched, some cushion and thermal and electrical insulation from the floor or ground on which it is laid. Both terms thermal and electrical insulation need to be clearly understood.

Almost all Yoga practices result in generation of thermal energy within your body during practice. Your body temperature is then different from the normal. This added heat does lots of good to your internal organs. You need to conserve and confine this thermal energy within your body during the practice sessions.

You also need to slowly and steadily release and discharge this energy during your relaxation phase. Once you understand all the basic principles of Yoga, you will know that most Yoga routines involve a stretch, hold, release and relax routine. All sessions must follow a relaxation phase compulsorily.

The duration of relaxation phase should be not less than thirty per cent of the time spent in practice sessions initially. It may be reduced to ten per cent after you master your craft. The thermal energy gained during practice gets released and the acquired incremental body temperature gets slowly dissipated and disappears during this relaxation phase. Any abrupt dissipation may be harmful. Therefore, the fabric and the clothing that you choose to lie down in, sit or stand for your practice sessions, must provide thermal insulation between your body and the floor/ground.

Similarly, during some of the practices your body gains static electricity. This added static electricity is also of immense value for your internal organs. Your nervous system works on a complex signal processing system. Many electrical signals in milli-Volts and nano-Amps range, regulate the functioning of the mind, heart and all other organs.

The Yogic practices by ways of generating static electricity in the desired manner, cause positive impacts on the nervous system, thus, affecting sets of emotions. Such static electricity also needs to be kept inside till it performs the desirable actions, and thereafter slowly discharged through the natural processes of your body. The surface during practise sessions should therefore provide electrical insulation.

The floor covering should also provide adequate cushion for your body. Some practices may require your complete body weight to rest and balance on few limbs. The fabric of the covering should be thick enough to provide cushion for comfort. Else, the limb holding your bodyweight may pain. In extreme cases, even injury may be caused. You may also keep a cushion handy to be used to support or provide relief to some organs, in cases of discomfort.

For those of you not endowed with technical knowledge of the subject, the above paragraphs may look a bit complex and intimidating. You may even be thinking of dropping the idea of further learning. Money is already wasted on the book, why waste more with so much of technical acquisitions involved. Well trust me! I am here to make your life simple.

You may actually pick up any old blanket, carpet or rug. It may even be tattered. Fold it in enough folds, such that the width is three times the width of your back. It should support your body while lying flat on your back with enough space to rotate your full body on right and left sides. Length should be enough to fit your body with arms fully stretched above your head. It should also provide good cushion. Thickness of more than 10 mm is good enough. Your Yoga mat is ready. Do remember to provide a clean absorbent cotton cloth to cover your Yoga mat. You may even reuse old discarded bed sheets after washing. You do not even have to make a trip to the market. You may start your practice sessions without making any more investments. You only need to invest time and patience.

You may, of course, use a Yoga mat commercially available in market, in attractive colours. Just get the dimensions right. Length should be near about the distance between your fingers and toes with your arms stretched upward pointing towards the sky. Width should be three times the width of your back. Thickness should not be less than 10 mm for proper cushioning.

You should keep handy a towel or a box of tissue papers to wipe sweat or nasal discharge. You may also keep a watch and a mirror as per your requirements. That is the complete set of tools and plants required for your practice.

To summarise, performing Yoga with a clean body, clean belly, clean mind, clean heart, and clean soul, in a neat and clean environment, shall give you best benefits and results.

Day-Three: Basics of Yoga: Part – II

Before We begin

In continuation of our yesterday's learning, we will learn some more basics of Yoga today.

Learning for the Day

Get Your Thought Process Right

This section may look a bit philosophical and boring to some of the readers. I have no intention of preaching morality and teaching philosophy to you. The problem is, Yoga does not work in isolation on your body. It doesn't involve your body alone. It involves more of your mind, your heart (signifying the set of emotions), and your soul (signifying your persona, aura, the halo around you).

The practices benefit your mind, heart and soul, more than your body. These complex correlations require some deeper understandings. You may be the enlightened one, knowing much more than me about these things. However, I am trying to be your teacher. It is my duty to tell you about these basics to make sure that your learning and your adoption of Yoga is smooth. So, kindly bear with me and hear me loud and clear!

Respect

The Nature

I assume that you have picked up this book, as you are an atheist, a rationalist, think more logically than the masses and have a scientific way of looking at things. You believe there is no God. Even if he/she exist, it is in forms and formats other than humans. You believe that the concept of God satisfies the following equations:

God = {Truth (The matrix and horizon of complete knowledge, ('Sampoorna Satya'))} Minus {Knowledge ('Jnana') (What is scientifically known and proven)}.

God = Set of Unknowns (The lack of knowledge, up to that time, about the origin, the purpose of life and universe and many other issues).

Many Yoga books and teachers preach spirituality. These books want you to say prayers to your creator, as if he/she is one to relish sycophancy, to be pleased and kept in good humour. They want you to thank him and be grateful to him. They profess to think about him, to be able to control your mind to meditate. In fact, this may be the most important factor for our resistance towards adoption of Yoga, so far.

I think you should have no problem, if I say that nature is your creator. It alone deserves all your praise, respect, regard and gratitude.

Nature encompasses the entire life support systems. It is the universe, the galaxies, the solar system, the sun, the moon, the earth, the air, the water, the beauty, the mighty mountains, the beautiful lakes, rivers, waterfalls, the seas, the humming birds and the bees, the flora and the fauna, the bio-diversity, the wide spectrum of life from tiny pollens, bacteria and viruses to the mighty elephants, tigers and lions. It also

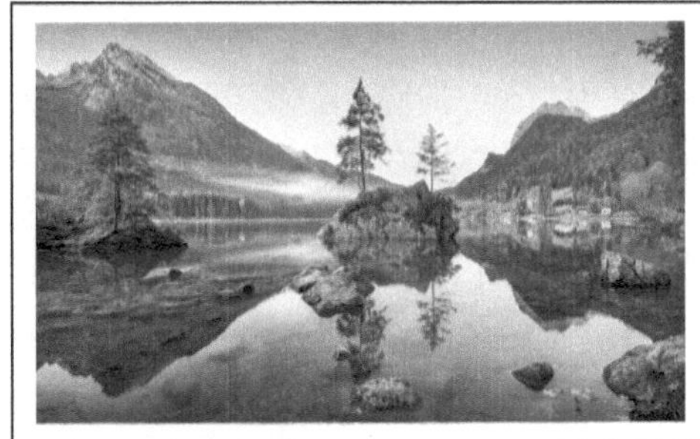

3.01: Respect the Nature

encompasses two most complex creations, the Man and the Woman. It has given you your life. Respect the nature.

The Government

Man is a social animal. The concept of life, without governance and without rule of law is still unimaginable. History tells us that civilisations survived and thrived under strong governments, where the rule of law prevailed. And empires vanished under weak kings.

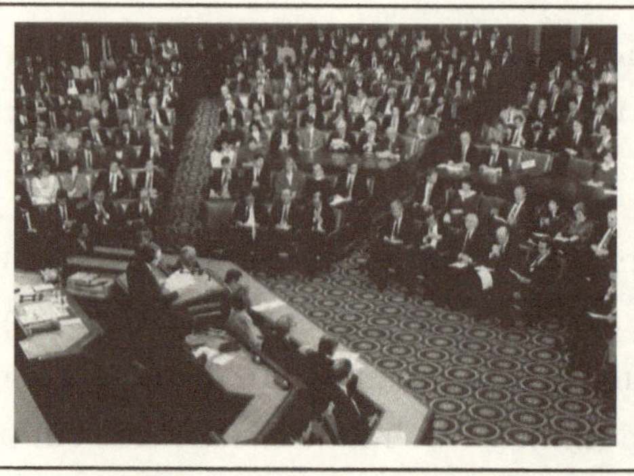

3.02: Respect Your Government

In ancient times, in the initial phases of evolution, the tribes were formed to unite people to enable them to fight united against wild animals, predators and adverse climates. Over the centuries the civilisations got matured and got organised into Village Panchayats (Local village level governments), Municipalities, Provincial and National Governments.

These systems have supported our lives. They are primarily responsible for your existence on this earth. The credits or discredits should therefore go more to them, than the artificial creator, elegantly housed in Mandir, Masjid, Gurudwara and Church. These institutions are serving the vested interests of a few greedy sections of society only.

That systems of governance are an unnecessary evil, in an ideal world, is another debate, best left out. You cannot have an ideal system. If there are no wild animals and predators in today's civilisation, man has assumed that role and filled the gap beautifully. He is the most dangerous predator. So, pay your taxes honestly and respect your Government.

The Society

The basic needs of life, food, clothing, housing, and reproduction (to satisfy the inbuilt zest for life) are beautifully fulfilled by nature, through a marvellous and complex eco-system. Humanity however, is not content and complete with these fulfilments. Humans have sets of complex emotions.

These emotions span a vast spectrum from absolute negatives to most positives. From greed to charity, from jealousy to competitive spirits, from hatred to love, compassion and respect, from ego, attitude, to humility and humbleness and the most beautiful emotion of love and desire to be loved.

The society fulfils all your needs, both positive and negative. Your inner circle of family and friends, your distant relatives, your lost friends—all provide you some ammunition to survive, thrive and carry on living. Can you imagine life devoid of all emotions? No? Okay! Therefore, the society deserves your respect and gratitude.

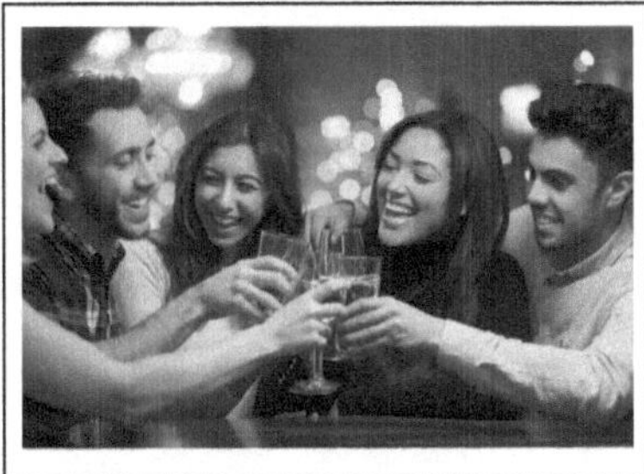

3.03: Respect the Society

We conveniently associate all emotions with the heart. In medical terms, the heart's sole purpose is to pump blood to various organs of your body. It is simply a pump with a set of valves, plungers and pistons. Even if you are a doctor and know the ins and outs of the heart, it is very convenient and useful to associate the complete set of human emotions with the heart.

So, when someone asks you to relax your heart, ask all your emotions of greed, lust, ego, jealousy, etc. to let go and relax. When you are commanded to control your emotions, do place a hand on your heart and say "Control," "Relax."

Similarly, it is convenient and useful to associate all your memories, intelligence, creativity and thinking with your mind. Let your knowledge that other parts of the body do contribute and complement such faculties, remain on back burner.

The Family

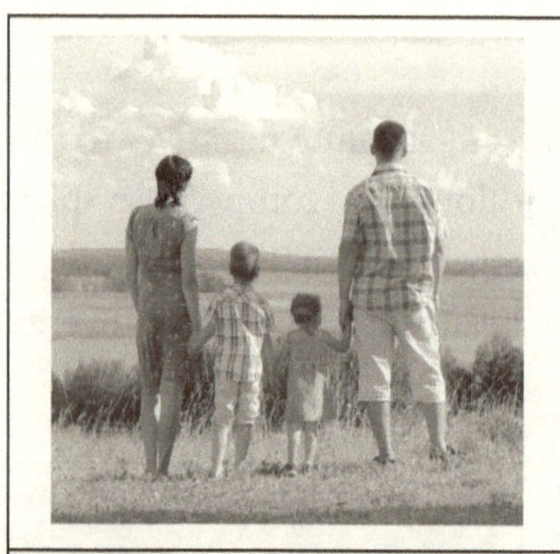

3.04: Respect Your Family

I shall be doing a disservice to your intelligence, if I need to remind you of the importance of your family in your life. Your parents, spouse, offspring, the near and the distant relatives, all are important. Only the degree of importance may vary. Doesn't your family deserve all the respect?

Yourself

Respect yourself. You are you. There is no one else like you. You are the unique creation of nature. There must be a unique purpose of nature behind your creation. You may or may not be aware of it, yet.

Love

I request you to simply read the above paragraphs by replacing respect/ gratitude with love. Love is the most beautiful human emotion. (I am repeating myself).

Understand

This is just a reminder. I do not wish to explain and elaborate. I assume you to have fantastic knowledge of these subjects. My only humble request is, read each sentence below as if chanting some 'mantra' loudly or silently in your mind, as it suits your fancy or style. Pause and ponder over the subject for a few minutes. Mull over whatsoever comes to your mind, before moving to the next sentence, the next mantra. Simple! Ok! Let's go!

Understand the Nature!

Understand the Nation!

Understand the Government!

Understand the society!

Understand the family!

Understand yourself!

Understand your body!

Understand your mind!

Understand the left hemisphere of your brain!

Understand the right hemisphere of your brain!

Understand your heart!

Understand your emotions!

Understand your personality!

Understand your persona!

Understand your aura!

Understand your soul!

Tired…? Okay!

Relax!… Relax!!…and… Relax!!!

The sole purpose of my boring lecture and the above bickering is to convince you that you and you alone are your sole creator. Everything else is a contributor, a catalyst and nothing else. Convinced! Okay! Let's summarise the learning of the days so far.

Table of the Day

Summary: Basics of Yoga practice			
When?	**Where?**	**How?**	**Wearing what?**
Early morning, before sunrise. Or Evening, no meals before and after.	Outdoor, neat and clean environment, fresh air. Or Indoor, neat and clean place.	Clean body, clean and hydrated belly. Clean mind. Sitting on a smooth surface, mat covered with absorbent cloth.	Minimum cotton, absorbent, loose clothes.

Channelize your mental energy: Get your thoughts right		
Respect	**Love**	**Understand**
The Nature	The Nature	The Nature
The Government	The Government	The Government
The Society	The Society	The Society
The Family	The Family	The Family
Yourself	Yourself	Yourself

Tutorials for the Day

1. Gather the basic information. When does the sun rise in your area? At what time do you usually get up from bed? Do you achieve a clean stomach effortlessly every day? Are you adequately hydrated during the day?

2. Chalk out your plans and strategy to achieve the objective of being able to spare a minimum of forty-five minutes for yourself. What behavioural changes are necessary?

3. Ponder over the question! What sets of emotions should your neighbour ideally have to make your life more comfortable, and peaceful? Do you possess this set of emotions? What changes are necessary in you, so that your neighbour considers you as an ideal neighbour?

4. Consciously observe your activities, your routine for the day. Is there any activity, just one single activity, that you can change for betterment of the nature and environment?

Day-Four: Basics of Yoga: Part – III

Learn before You Leap

Let us continue from where we left yesterday and learn a few more basics of Yoga.

Learning for the Day

Enjoy Everything

You must enjoy, rejoice, and feel happy at every step of your learning process. You must also enjoy all your practice sessions. And most important, you should enjoy imbibing Yoga in life. Many exercises shall ask you for deep breathings, forceful exhalation, stretching your limbs and rotating them. Perform all such steps in smooth, flowing-like-water, dance-like movements manner, feeling happy about it, enjoying it.

Do not over stretch any part of your body beyond your capacity to feel happy about stretching it. Feel pressures and pleasures, not pain! Stop immediately, if you feel any discomfort, any pain, and immediately go to the relaxation phase/posture. For this, it is important that you understand the relaxation posture associated with each of the exercise postures. Pay specific attention to the topic during your learning of the day in Chapter-One, Day-Six to Day-Nine.

During all your practices and after regular daily exercise, do make it a habit to ask yourself, "How did I feel?" Reply honestly. If your answer is anything other than good or okay, stop practice! Give yourself a break! Try again, if you really feel like it.

Count Everything

Make it a habit to count everything. Everything! Howsoever mundane or nonsensical it may look like, initially. Count the number of pages that you have read so far. Minutes spent in reading them. Many of the exercises shall require that you count your breathings. Do it honestly.

A few exercises may require you to repeat a set of motions for a fixed number of times. It shall help if you are counting, else may result into overdoing and unnecessarily tiring yourself. Not completing the set of exercises properly, for lack of counting, may also not be desirable.

Counting also helps you in improving your concentration, in channelizing your mental energy the way you want it to be. These techniques play a very crucial role in meditation, one of the most important components of Yoga. Channelizing and regulating all your internal (Mind, Metabolism, Electrical, etc.) and external (Physical) energies in a planned manner, is what distinguishes Yoga from other forms of exercises.

You may be wondering, how does one count breathing. Well it depends on you. Your breathing actually is completed in three steps. Taking air in (inhalation), keeping the air inside body (retention), and allowing air to exit your body (exhalation). You may count the complete set of inhalation, retention and exhalation as one breath. Or else you may count inhalation and exhalation separately. Try it. Observe what you are comfortable with and follow the same system for all that you're counting. By the way, do not forget the multiplication by two required, if your instructor asks you to complete ten sets of breathings and you are counting inhalation and exhalation separately. In that case you are required to count up to twenty to complete ten sets of breathings.

Time Everything

You should time everything. Mentally make note of time spent on each activity. It shall be best if you may mentally set a target for the time frame, before commencing any activity. After completion compare actual time spent with pre-set target. In case of vast variations, ponder over the questions. Was the target wrong? Or did you need to hurry up or slow down during actions?

During practice sessions and your daily Yoga routine sessions, it should make sense to keep a watch handy near your mat, if outdoors. If indoor, you may place a wall clock easily visible from your place of practice. You may fix a time frame (minimum forty-five minutes) and a set of exercises to be completed during the session. Compare after completion of time or set and take corrective measures for next sessions.

One word of caution! Do not form the habit of looking at the watch after completing every small activity. Do not search for the watch every minute. This will cause unnecessary distractions. Your mind must concentrate on, be focussed, be devoted and dedicated and be at the sole discretion of the activity at hand. Mind is a wild aimless wanderer. It is a habitual multi-tasker. It is very difficult to tame it and keep it at one place. But that is what you must do to achieve best results. So, time everything, frequently using your inbuilt sense of timing, your biological clock and rarely using the external clock.

Tip of the Day

Tip: Instant Nourishment
If you feel weak and exhausted, before, during and immediately after your Yoga practice, you may consume small amount of honey in lukewarm water for instant hydration, nourishment and energy.

Synchronise Everything

You need to harmonise and synchronise a lot of things in life. But in Yoga, you need to primarily synchronise, three things—actions, breaths, and thoughts. This on the face of it looks very easy, but one needs to put in sustained efforts and practise regularly to achieve this. When you achieve harmony in these three, the three sources of energy complement each other. You derive the best benefits even with, as routine an exercise as, breathing normally. The synchronisation between mind (thoughts) and actions is easy to understand, but difficult to achieve. This, you will achieve with routine practices only. Let us tackle the easier subject first, i.e., achieving coordination between actions/exercises and breathings.

Most Yogic routines invariably specify the two issues, namely, place where mind and thoughts are to be focussed, and the correct way of breathing while performing the routine. There are specific instructions on these aspects. If there is no specific instruction, the breathing is to be regulated as under:

- **Inhale:** When bending, tilting or moving upper body in front directions. Whenever stretching your body in upwards directions. When tilting or taking body to left/right directions from central position.

- **Exhale:** When bending, tilting, moving upper body in backward direction. Whenever releasing stretch from body and bringing it in downward directions. When de-tilting or moving body from left/right directions to the centre.

- **Retain:** When holding on to any posture.

- In the Stretch-Hold-Release-Relax routines, breathing is to follow a perfectly timed and synchronised Inhale-Retain-Exhale-Breathe normally pattern.

- In routines involving rotations, synchronise the breathings, i.e., complete one breathing with one rotation.

The Yogic routines do also invariably specify the action/activity/body-organ/point where attention of mind and senses is to be focussed. Please note carefully that instruction shall invariably ask you to focus 'attention' or focus 'mind.' This focus however is not limited to attention of mind; it also includes focus of all your senses. As you are aware, there are five basic senses and correspondingly five sensory organs. These are, touch (fingertips and many other organs), vision (eyes), smell (nose), sound (ears), and taste (mouth/tongue). It is believed that a sixth sense of intuition too is there. In Yoga, you have the liberty to keep this at rest. But, all five basic senses need to be focussed, as instructed.

If the instructions are silent about the activity/point of focus, this focus is to be maintained at 'focal point of all senses.' I will subsequently elaborate on this point. This, 'the focal point of all senses' is the 'default option' for focus.

Music and Yoga

Most text books on Yoga recommend performing exercises in a silent environment. Sounds of all types are considered distractions and obstruction for attaining focus of mind. I, however find the environment more conducive with a soft music playing in the background. It actually depends on personal choice. If you are a music enthusiast, you are more likely to enjoy your Yoga with some music of your liking. Conduct your own experimentations and observations and decide yourself. Do not get bogged down by the logic of silence being the best for concentration and focus.

Music may also help you in timing your actions and sessions. You generally know the timing of a song or track playing in the background. If you are stuck on one exercise for the full length of track, whereas it should have taken you just half the track length, you know it is time to leave and move on to the next set of exercises.

Achieving concentration and focus of your mind (signifies the thought processes and the thinking subconsciously going on in your mind) and heart (signifies your set of emotions) also gets facilitated with music since there is a second reference point available in music. Your thoughts are likely to waver and go to music. Your heart may abort the task at hand, but is likely to get trapped in the emotions of music. It is easier to pull back your mind and heart from this reference point (music) back to the task at hand. In silence, you never know where these two will find solace and rest.

Music and Yoga have many other similarities also, some of which deserve your attention and understanding.

- A perfect arrangement of sound is music; rest is cacophony. A perfect set of exercise to suit your body, mind, heart and soul is Yoga; rest is exercise in futility.

- Synchronisation of various sounds emanating from vocal chords and various musical instruments is music. Yoga encourages you to build similar synchronisation in your life. Your body, mind, heart and soul achieve perfect harmony and synchronisation. The various energies within your body also get synchronised and harmonised. The balances, the control and regulatory systems, all get synchronised.

- Smooth flow of sound is music. Transition from one note to another is always soft. During Yogic practices all movements of your body, your breathing must also flow smoothly. All transitions from one posture to another must be musically smooth. No jerks and no abrupt throws. Everything must be soft and smooth.

- Music touches your heart and your mind. It provides solace, peace, comfort and energy. It refreshes your mind. So, does Yoga.

Dance and Yoga

Are you a dancer? All of us are. Good or bad; doesn't matter! Even if you can't dance, you must have enjoyed some good dance performances. If you haven't seen a dance performance recently, I request you to keenly, carefully and observantly watch a few dance performances. Particularly, those dance forms where the finger formations, hand gestures, the facial expressions, and bodily expressions are important, like 'Bharatnatayam' and 'Katthak'

(Indian classical dance forms). Also, those dance forms, where the upward stretching of upper torso, spinal movements and feet or toe tapping are given primacy. Closely observe the following:

- Use of the thumb, fingers and palms in formation of various hand gestures, each conveying a different expression and meaning.

- Spine straight, spine stretched upward, complete upper body rotating or moving smoothly, supported on spine alone.

- Toes pointed.

- Foot or toe tapping.

Each of these observations shall be very helpful in your further learning and understandings. And man! Let me assure you that you definitely will be a better dancer after you adopt Yoga.

Storytelling and Yoga

Have you thought of or tried story-writing as a career option? No? You must at least be a good story-teller. There is a story-writer, a story-teller, hidden within all of us, yelling for freedom. All of us need this skillset sometimes to entertain kids or some other times to get out of stickier situations with wife or boss.

Well there are marked similarities in Storytelling and Yoga too. Am I taking the things too far? Not really! Read on!

In many breathing exercises ('Pranayama'), subtle exercises ('Sukshma-Vyayaam') and Yogic exercises ('Yoga Asanas') you will be asked to practice, perform and repeat a specific set of practices with varying degrees of difficulties. In your routine daily practices also, it is desirable that a few Asanas, having at least three to four variations in difficulty levels are performed repeatedly (may be for ten or more counts).

Under such situations, you are likely to be confused. Which is to be performed first, and which later? Difficult one goes first or later? It is best to fall back upon your knowledge of storytelling, in such situations.

Each story has a build-up phase, where you introduce characters, identify protagonist, villains, assign them characters and build up the plot. The story thereafter traverses towards the climax, where the narrative reaches a peak. The story finally has an ending with a 'and they lived happily thereafter' or some similar tagline.

You are advised to decide the pace, the difficulty level arrangements, like a story. Start slow, then let there be a build-up phase, reach crescendo in middle, slow down and end on a slow and happy note.

Are some sinister ideas suggesting to me that I could have explained it better with some other analogy running in your mind? Man! You are naughty!

Left Is Right, or Right Is Right?

Some of the subtle exercises, Pranayama and Yoga Asanas may require you to perform a set of routines first with one of your limbs (hand, leg, foot, nostril, etc.) and later with second limb. Sometimes, it may be first limb, second limb, and both limbs together routine. You may get confused, which limb goes first, left or right? There are many other issues your poor brain must monitor. You may end up doing the routine twice using right or left limb only. Therefore, the question, which goes first, must be properly answered, understood and adopted.

Answer is quite simple. If you are a right-hander, left goes first and vice-versa. Explanation is also simple. Your reflexes will prompt you to start with right, till brain detects and warns you. When you are starting you are relying more on brain. During the routine, you are more at the mercy of your reflexes.

Eyes Shut or Open?

Conventional text books on the subject prescribe to keep the eyes closed, for facilitating focus and attention. However, in the initial phase of your learning, it is important that you see and observe your actions. So that you may compare and check, "was it the way you learnt it, and wanted it to be?" It therefore should make sense to keep the eyes open, in the initial phases. Once you gain reasonable proficiency, you should keep the eyes closed. In Meditation and Pranayama, it is better that eyes remain perfectly shut.

Mirrors Don't Lie

For smoothening your learning process, let me give you one more important hint. If practising indoors, you may use a frameless, full length mirror (height of the mirror should be greater than half of your height from toe to tips of fingers, with hands placed upwards over your head, fingers pointing towards the sky) placed slightly inclined with a wall for support. This is so that you may observe your full body, all your actions and movements. This way you can observe if your movements/actions are smooth and in the same way as was prescribed.

Focal Point of Your Senses (इन्द्रियों का केंद्रबिंदु ॥)

Meditation (ध्यान) and breathing exercises (प्राणायाम) are two very important component of Yoga. Both require control, regulation, coordination and synchronisation of your brain activities, breathing activities and control of all your senses. Close your eyes and you may control your vision. Sit in silence and your hearing senses are under your control. Your nose as such is busy tasked with taking care of your breathing, so controlling sense of smell is also not a problem. The problem is mind and emotions. Acquiring absolute control over them and channelizing their energies is a tedious issue.

Yoga has the solution. Ask your brain and your heart to focus on the 'focal point of all your senses.' So, you will be asked to focus on the focal point of your senses. Now your first need is to find where this point is.

If you observe closely, the majority of your sensory organs are located on the top storey of your body, above your neck.

If you observe closely, the centre of gravity of your head will perhaps lie beneath a point between your eyes. A point at which your two eyebrows meet to have a rendezvous. It is just above your nose line, with the tip of your nose observing and guarding this point. If you are blessed with a nice round face, chances are that this point is at the centre of a circle representing your face. Could you find it? Now give a gentle massage on the point and surroundings. How does it feel?

To focus your attention (mind) and all senses on this point, you may initially develop a routine. Consciously ask your brain that some important activity, some pleasant vibrations are soon going to happen at this point. Ask your brain to be observant and wait for this activity. Simultaneously, tell your nose that some very pleasant smell will soon emanate from this point, and he must be attentive and wait for this pleasing odour. Pass similar commands to the touch organs, taste organs and ears. Tempting them for a pleasing-healing touch, some mouth-watering taste and the most beautiful music…

Believe me, if you achieve a perfect focus of mind and senses on this focal point, while chanting 'Aum,' you may sometimes(rarely) experience all these organs reporting back to you, that all these 'pleasant-vibrations,' 'pleasing-odour,' 'pleasing-healing-touch,' 'mouth-watering-taste' and 'most-beautiful-musical-sounds' actually happened.

So, do not get carried away if someone tells you that he had a 'divine experience,' 'got one-to-one with God' or 'got united with the creator.' You now know, what it really was. There is hardly anything in Yoga beyond the unification of all energies and the phenomenon of resonance in all these 'out of this world experiences' aggressively sold for marketing purposes. Try and experience it yourself, before some 'Guru' gives you this divine experience and creates a big dent on your 'atheism.' I shall henceforth be referring to this point as 'focal point.'

Food

Most text books on Yoga recommend vegetarian diet as ideal for Yoga practices and Yogic way of life. This is expected. All religions of the continent, particularly Jainism, Buddhism and Hinduism preach vegetarianism as best dietary habits. Vegetarianism is also associated with 'Ahimsa' (Non-Violence), a concept believed, preached and propagated by the idols and the icons of the Indian continent.

Non-violence was the central point of Buddha's preaching and Mahatma Gandhi's philosophy. It is also believed that vegetarian dietary habits ensure that body and mind are flexible and well prepared for Yogic practice.

However, your dietary preferences should in no way hamper your acceptance and adoption of Yoga. I urge you to start your practice without changing your dietary habits. You are also encouraged to conduct experimentation on yourself. Believe me, that is the best way to find out what suits you the best, rather than believing the text books or me.

After your learning phase is over, do try both diets for a fixed number of days, say fifteen to thirty days. Your dietary preferences should, in any case, be not so rigid to make survival difficult, without your favourite pound of flesh for fifteen to thirty days. Observe how you feel in both the phases. Decide for yourself!

While on food, let me remind you of the precaution. Do not consume any solid food at least forty-five minutes before practice. Food should be consumed only twenty to thirty minutes after the practice.

Do-It-Yourself or Learn from 'Guru'/Teacher/Instructor?

This is the trickiest question. Pick up any book on Yoga, you will surely find one Chapter or at least one paragraph, devoted to the importance of teacher/trained instructor/experts. Most text books/teachers advise learning only from an instructor. Do-it-yourself is not an option, deserving of even consideration.

A few books take the subject to extremes. Epitomes are written to warn you not to attempt any Yogic practice, any Pranayama, and any Asana, except under close supervision of an expert. As if heavens will fall on you if you are just doing 'kapalabhati' without paying fee to a teacher. Please understand, that in ancient times, the times when Yoga originated and evolved, there were hardly any means of communications.

There were limitations of language, printing, photography, audio and video recordings. And of course, there was no internet, no Smartphone, no Google, and no YouTube. The only available mode of communication, in those times was oral instructions from teacher ('Guru') to disciple ('Shishya').

Some of the Yogic practices are complex, some may cause harm if not performed properly, and some definitely are dangerous. The best option available in those times, to safeguard the health and wellbeing of disciples, was to stipulate that all learning and practice will take place under supervision of a teacher.

This cardinal principle stipulated in ancient texts is still being followed and reproduced. There is a commercial advantage in keeping the principle intact, even in modern times.

I however beg to differ. The teacher is important. His importance lies in leading you, guiding you, informing you the precautionary measures and the possible dangers. He is required to take care of your health and wellbeing.

But he is required, only if you are not capable of doing it yourself. If you can read books, assimilate the information and knowledge, understand the precautions and associated dangers, validate and cross-check the differing information from diverse sources, then you do not need a teacher. All you need is the information, the correct and accurate information.

And herein lies the problem. The problem is, Yoga is an assimilated science. It is a carefully crafted package from different sources, in different times. There are many types, many schools of Yoga. Some are orthodox, traditional, staunch believers in ancient versions, and in puritan and pure form of Yoga. Some are modern, progressive, are open to experimentations, new additions and deletions. A clear majority lies in between the two extremes. All have the same Yoga at the core, at their helm. There are variations in methods, intensity and the way of teaching. But chances are, if you gather information about one technique from three sources, you may get three different versions of information.

And therefore, herein lies the answer to the basic query. Do-it-yourself OR learn from Guru/Teacher/Instructor? The answer lies within you. If you can gather information from four to five different credible sources, assimilate the information, tie up the loose ends, smoothen the sharp edges and pointed corners, find a middle path in contradictions and decide best fit for you, then 'Do-It-Yourself' is the best path for you. Even if you go to a teacher, you may soon discover that doing it yourself was better. Learning on your own, gives better rewards than relying on the limited knowledge of a teacher. If you are not the exploration, experimentation, adoption type, going to a teacher is better for you.

No matter whichever path you take, remember the golden rules.

1. Better safe than sorry. Understand the precautions first; even before reading, seeing or learning about a practice, learn the precautions. By the way, let me share with you, that I also learnt a very important lesson of book writing, while telling you this. I shall be writing precautions before the description of practice/Asana.

2. Learn before you leap. Gather information from at least five different credible sources and from different mediums such as Print, Photographs, Internet, Video, Apps, Smartphone; explore everything and gather as much as you may assimilate, depending upon your appetite and aptitude. Understand different versions, different variations, and different difficulty levels of the same practice. Decide your best fit. Start practice with your best fit. Experiment, explore, learn and change later.

3. Attention to precautions/intimidations should be commensurate with the difficulty level. For meditative postures, easier breathings, subtle exercises not involving too much of stretching, too much of pressure and forces, just do not bother much, if you are healthy. Even if you do not do it the perfect way, no harm is caused. Only for complex, complicated exercises (explicitly marked as difficult) precautions are important.

Last but Not the Least

For adoption of Yoga in your life, for your basic learning, this DIY guide is sufficient. You need not bother much about other issues. Just follow the instructions.

Relax…! Relax…!! and… Relax!!!

Now that you have carefully gone through and assimilated the above contents, you only need to learn some more of precautions and some postures to be ready to start your practice sessions. Precautions shall form part of the learning for day-five. We will start learning posture from day-six.

Tutorials for the Day

Do the following honestly and diligently during the day.

1. Imagine that someone asks you to thank or remember your creator. What is the first thing that comes to your mind? What all comes to your mind? Write down in one paragraph, without pretending to be what you are not!

2. Sit comfortably in any posture and count your breaths up to twenty inhalations and exhalations, breathing slowly.

3. If you have a desk job, requiring long hours of sitting, leave your desk at every two hours interval, walk twenty steps.

If possible raise your hands one at a time and tilt your body to the left slightly, while raising right hand and vice-versa. Repeat a few times.

4. At least once during the day, close your eyes, sitting or standing in any comfortable posture, close your ears by gentle pressure of your thumb, breath slowly, without using any force for exhalation or inhalation. Let your brain focus on the point between your eyebrows and above the starting point of nose (focal point). Count to fifty. Observe how you felt after this.

Day-Five: Basics of Yoga: Part – IV

Preliminary Precautions

Learning for the Day

I shall now be summarising and reiterating the preliminary precautions that you must observe, before you start your practice. Some of them may be a mere repetition. Repetition is deliberate.

You need to understand that these precautions form the core of all Yogic practices. You, in fact, need to inculcate the habit of mentally making a check list without using pen and paper, the sticky notes, and the Smartphone. You need to develop the habit of checking, rechecking and cross checking all your actions, movements, and sessions with this check list. And mind it! You must do it without allowing your mind to drift away. You need to do this, while concentrating on the task at hand, without losing the focus.

Remember my advice in 'How to use this guide' section. Before starting actual practices, you must know your vital health statistics, the key health indicators and parameters (the physical attributes). If you haven't got your routine medical examination done in the recent past (say last six months), it is time to visit the hospital or your general physicians for routine medical check-up. Particularly, you must know your height, weight, BMI, Blood Pressures (BP), Blood sugar levels, Heart beat rate, Spinal and heart conditions.

These precautions are given here in point form for easy reference and recollection. Credit for inspiration in writing this section goes to the publication titled "International Day of Yoga, 21st June,

Common Yoga Protocol" by Government of India, Ministry of Ayurveda, Yoga & Naturopathy, Unani, Siddha and Homoeopathy.

Before the Practice

- Cleanliness is an important prerequisite for Yogic practice. It includes cleanliness of surroundings, air, body, mind, thoughts and emotions.

- Yogic practices are recommended to be performed in a calm and quiet atmosphere, with a relaxed body and mind. You may, if it suits you, play some soft music in the background. If you cannot find such a calm and quiet place, you need to train your ears to hear only pleasant sounds and be not receptive to the cacophony, the noise or any other disturbing, distracting sounds. Believe me your mind and ears can achieve it, you only need to cajole and guide your hearing systems.

- Yogic practice should be done on empty stomach or light stomach. This is important to achieve concentration. This is also important as many Yogic practices have a cleansing and cleaning effect on your internal organs. If you have ever washed or dry cleaned your clothes, you would know that cleaning is best achieved if the clothes were previously reasonably clean. It is difficult to wash a dirty cloth. You require lots of detergent. This in turn causes lots of water pollution. You also harm the water bodies, where the effluent water after cleaning is discharged.

- Bladder and bowels should be empty before starting Yogic practices.

- You may use a thin mattress (not the ones having springs, not more than 20 mm thick), Yoga mat, (ideally 10–20 mm thick), durries, rug, carpet, or folded blanket for your practice. This should provide both thermal and electrical insulation. Cover your mat with cotton absorbent sheet for allowing sweat to dissipate. You may keep a towel or box of tissue papers, a cushion and a watch handy.

- Light and comfortable cotton clothes facilitate smooth and easy movements of body and parts.

- Yoga should not be performed in a state of exhaustion, illness, in a hurry, or in acute stress conditions. Do not practise after spending sizable time under the hot sun. Do not practise outdoors when the sun is hot and fuming.

- You must consult a physician, or a Yoga therapist, if suffering from any chronic disease/pain/cardiac problems, before the practice.

- (For girls) A general physician or Yoga expert should be consulted before doing Yogic practices during pregnancy and menstruation.

During the Practice

- Practice sessions should start with a prayer, a positive-auto-suggestion, a chant, or invocation. This creates a conducive environment to relax the mind. This also creates a positive energy.

- The practices shall be performed slowly, in a relaxed manner, with awareness of the body and breath. The body movements need to be synchronised and harmonised with breathing and focus of mind.

- Do not unnecessarily hold your breath. Hold it only if specifically mentioned/instructed to do so. While holding breath, keep on mentally counting the numbers, preferably at the rate of one per second, to keep track of time. Release retention of breath at the slightest hint of discomfort.

- Breathing should be always through the nostrils, unless mentioned/instructed otherwise. The computer/processor in your brain must be configured to treat nostrils as the 'default option' for breathing.

- Do not hold the body tightly, unless instructed, or jerk the body abruptly at any point of time.

- While standing and sitting for practice, the spine/backbone should be straight and upright and not bent, curved or drooping.

- Perform the practice according to your own capacity. Do not unnecessarily compete with others, particularly with the younger and healthier lots. Remember you are not here for exhibition of your physical prowess.

- It generally takes significant time to master the art, and the practices to show the results. So, be persistent and patient. Sustained continuation of practices is very essential.

- There are contra-indications/limitations for each Yoga practice and such contra-indications should be well understood and kept in mind.

- Yoga session should also end with proper relaxation phase and some prayers, positive-auto-suggestion, meditation, deep silence or chanting for world/humanity peace. Remember to pace your session akin to a story, i.e., a happy ending story. Allow all the villains to die and all protagonist/supporting casts and characters to lead a happy healthy life, thereafter. Peace, health and happiness shall automatically come to you.

After Practice

- After the exercise, massage ankles, calf muscles and knees, gently, uniformly but firmly to derive optimum results.

- Bath should be taken only after twenty to thirty minutes of practices. Give your body some well-deserved rest for twenty to thirty minutes. Remember, you need to allow smooth, gradual dissipation of excess thermal, electrical and other energies gained.

- Food should be consumed only after twenty to thirty minutes of practices.

Assimilate and understand the above points carefully. Prepare your check list, even if you need to use pen and paper, or Smartphone initially. Continue, if everything is as per check list. If not, stop, ponder, make corrections and continue thereafter.

I shall be routinely writing 'Follow the prerequisites' in the first few days of learning in this and subsequent chapters. This is to remind you the prerequisites for achieving the best results for your practice. The prerequisites that are being referred to in the phrase are the ones that have been taught in the learning so far. The subject of Day-One to Day-Five learning shall henceforth be referred to as 'Follow the prerequisites.' Do remember to run through your own check list.

Tutorial for the Day

1. During the day time, whenever you find some spare time, try and recollect the precautions and instructions you learnt today, without referring to this guide or any other book/other tools. Make a list in point form. Count how many points/issues you can recollect. Later compare your list and count with the points/issues in this section. Your ideal score is twenty-four. You are ready for starting your practice, if you score above twenty. Else, kindly go through the contents once again.

Day-Six: The Yogic Postures: Part – I
Basics and Hands Formations (HASTA-MUDRA)

Learning for the Day

We shall now be learning some Yoga postures, the poses that you need to attain to start the Yogic practices. But first it is important to understand what a 'Yoga posture' is.

Comfortably positioning the body, with joy, in some specific posture, holding it there, for some specified durations, with full concentration of mind over certain body parts, and controlling breathings, as directed, is the 'Yoga posture.' Please re-read this definition slowly and understand the meanings of all phrases.

Most Yogic exercises are performed in any one of the following poses:

- Sitting on the mat, with legs in front or folded in some specific manner (Sitting Posture).

- Standing on your legs, toes, heels, hands, arms or head (Standing posture).

- Lying down on your back (Supine posture) or belly (Prone posture).

For all these exercises, there is a starting pose. First attain this pose, relax and then perform tips and turns movements, rotations, as instructed. Recollect the Stretch-Hold-Release-Relax routines. For each set of exercises, there is a relaxation pose.

You need to go to this pose in your relaxation phase after completing prescribed routine, or at first hint of tiredness, pain, fatigue or breathlessness. Invariably, the starting pose is also the relaxation pose. Before starting any routine, you must clearly understand the relaxation posture that you need to migrate to in emergencies. 'Shavasana' is the 'default option' for all relaxation needs.

Some Basics First

Spine Straight

1. Positioning of spine in all postures is very important. Unless instructed otherwise, spine must be straight. Straight means slightly stretched upwards, in a straight line and perpendicular to the ground when standing or sitting. When lying down, in supine or prone posture, it must be a straight line parallel to the ground. Do not bend, or allow any sagging or loosening of your spine, unless instructed to do so, for a specific exercise and for a specific duration.

2. It will do you lots of good in life if you inculcate the habit of keeping the spine straight in everyday life also. While sitting, standing, climbing and getting down stairs, check spine straight, correct and move. Make it a habit.

Head Held High

Head should be resting straight upwards on shoulders and neck. Neckline and spine should be in straight lines. Weight of head should be smoothly transferring from neck to spine, spine to legs, and from legs to ground. Transfer of weight from upper to lower body should also be smooth and straight.

Line of vision must be straight, parallel to ground, eyes focussed on an object placed at infinite distance at the same height as yours. In day-to-day life also always walk with head held high. Talk to your boss and wife with head held high. You will either be fired/divorced, or your respect will increase many folds. Take the risk. Unless instructed to relax and loosen up, neck should be slightly stretched upwards.

Toes Pointed

Remember the 'Dance and Yoga' section in earlier parts of learning. You were encouraged to understand the importance of 'pointed toes' in dance. Mild stretching outwards applied on toes to pull the muscle and associated nerve system, connecting feet with upper parts of body and the brain is important in many Yogic postures. Unless asked to 'relax the toes,' toes should always be in pointed state. So, the 'default option' for 'toes positioning' is 'stretched outwards and pointed.'

Just in case you encounter some difficulty in understanding the concepts thus far, the stepwise procedure is as under:

- Follow the prerequisites.

- Stand upright on your legs, hands hanging loosely by the side of your body, riveted on shoulders, palms loose, and fingers pointing downwards.

- Now give your neck a slight upward stretch without jerks, as if trying to add a few millimetres to your apparent height. You may use power of your breath by preceding the action with one deep inhalation. Release the breath, and hold neck and head in the same position, i.e., stretched slightly upward.

- Now also give your upper body a gentle upward stretch, using power of your breath with deep inhalation without jerks. You may use the powers of muscles in your belly by an inward squeeze.

- Make a conscious effort to add a few more millimetres to your apparent height by raising your full body upward, pointing toes, stretching arms downwards, tucking belly inside, expanding chest and uniformly balancing the body weight on toes and heels. Check that spine-line and neckline are together plotting a straight line or making an angle, as close to 180 degrees as possible, at spine-hip joint. Breathe normally holding this posture.

You may better appreciate the importance of the 'Spine straight, head held high' concept with an example.

Suppose you must face an important selection (say, in the Army). The selection is important to you, your career, and your future. There is a rigid pre-set criterion of meeting certain height for selection. You are just meeting the criteria marginally.

Your selection depends on the way measurements are taken. If found slightly shorter during measurements, you may face rejection. The way you will stand facing the measurement wall, in your desperation to add those few millimetres to your height, is the way to follow for this concept. This is also the pathway to improve your 'body language' in everyday life.

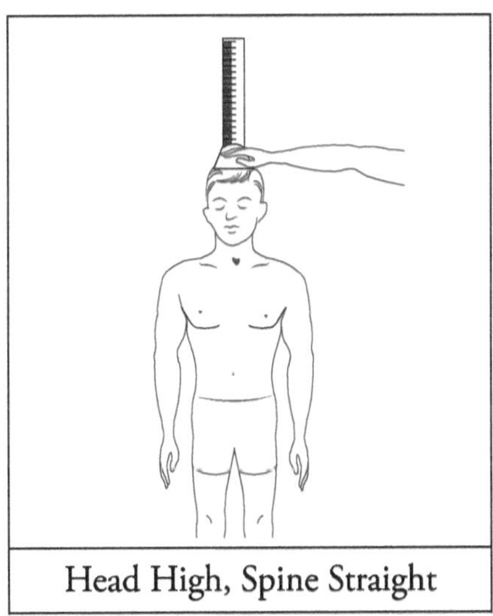

Head High, Spine Straight

Hand Formations. HASTA-MUDRA (हस्तमुद्रा)

Hands are very important. After all, they perform all your tasks. They take so much care of the other organs of your body. You also should take special care of them during exercises. They need to be involved adequately in all exercises.

The hand formations, the way you place your thumbs and hand fingers, the way you create some pressure on certain points in your hand, palm and fingertips, the way you rub and massage these points, enhances the benefits of the Yogic practices.

The statement that a mere bending and pressing of fingers, making some formations using thumbs, fingers and palm, or mere exertion of some pressure on some pores in hand, or merely massaging some tissues, may have some impact on mind, heart, and on the diseases and ailments of body, may not be very palatable to your logical and scientific mind. Detailed logical and scientific explanation for this is available.

You invariably use your fingertips to gauge the hotness or coldness, i.e., the relative temperature of water. You may also use other organs, such as toes, palm, for the same activity. Results, as you know, may or may not be the same. There are receptors in your fingertips, and other organs to feel (not measure) the temperature of water.

There is a signal processing mechanism to tell your brain the relevant information that it asked for. Is the water hot, or cold? Or hotter/colder than expected? If you deliberately assign this task of sensing hotness/coldness of water, to the toes, instead of fingertips, the information to the brain may be different. This means your fingertips and adjoining organs in hands are relatively better placed than other organs to directly communicate with brain.

Yogic postures, as you know, require you to 'relax the brain,' 'focus' and 'keep attention pointed.' For this you need to constantly communicate with the brain.

So, when you need a good, reliable and direct channel of communication with brain, what can be better than this channel? All that you are required to do is to fold the fingers in some specific manners, apply some pressures in specified manners, massage and caress a few tissues, cause mild piercing action with nails, and you can send signals to your brain. Now create some variations and some codes and you have a language ready for secret communications, between hands and mind.

Another explanation for the importance of hands formations lies in 'energy block principles.' You know that your body is dissipating heat.

The sensors in those automatic gates that open on your approach sense this body heat dissipation. Heat is the lowest form of energy.

Your body also radiates and dissipates many other energies. The escape gates for these leakages of energies are in various organs, primary ones being in hands and feet. 'Yogic-mudra' is an art of putting some locks on these porous gates, blocking these energy leakages, radiations and dissipations. Thus, these energies are redirected and re-channelized back to body for doing some more good work.

This, in a nutshell is what 'Yogic Hasta-Mudra' is. For ease of acceptance and understanding you may look at it as a language for communication between brain and its trusted transducers for regulating energy flows in your body. The 'Hand Mudras' otherwise are believed to impact your body, your mind, your heart and the bodily disease and disorders. Herein lies the beauty of Yoga. It has actually created a package involving all organs, all actions to aid and abet each other. You should learn the following hand formations carefully.

1. Hand Formation for Salutation: ('NAMASKAR MUDRA')

Steps:

- Follow the prerequisites.

- Sit or stand in any comfortable position. Hands loosely hung by the side.

- Fold your right arm and bring it in front, palm facing on left side, fingers closed (joined together), place your hand on your chest, tips of fingers touching the bottom of chin.

- Now fold your left arm, palm facing rightwards, and join both palms. Hold both palms together tightly, tips of fingers of both hands touching the bottom of chin.

- This is the hand posture for Salutation 'The Namaskar Mudra.'

2. Hand Formation for Knowledge and Consciousness: 'JNANA MUDRA' and 'CHIN MUDRA'

Steps:

- Follow the prerequisites.

- Sit or stand in any comfortable position. Hands loosely hung by the side.

- Stretch your hand outward, feeling mild tension on your shoulder joints, keeping elbow straight. Stretch all your fingers and thumbs outward keeping five to ten millimetres gap between fingers feeling some pressure, some extra rush of blood and some reddening in your palm. Now close your fist tightly keeping thumb enveloped in rest of four fingers. Release the fist. Repeat this set for four to five times. This way, you warm up your palm.

- Now bend your index fingers and allow it to gently press your thumbs, the fingers and thumb forming a circle, tip of finger should be exerting mild pressure on top of thumb. Top of thumb should also be exerting equal pressure on tip of index finger. Middle finger, ring finger and little finger, remaining slightly stretched, close to each other. Place the hand on the knees with palms facing downwards. This gesture, this hand formation is beneficial for your mind. This is called Jnana mudra. It is believed to provide knowledge and facilitate concentration.

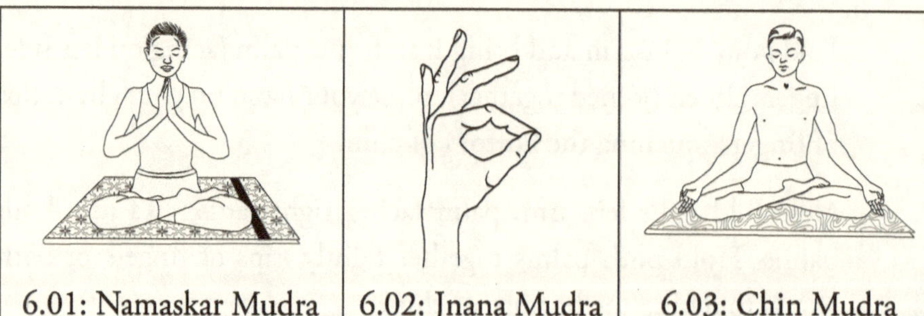

| 6.01: Namaskar Mudra | 6.02: Jnana Mudra | 6.03: Chin Mudra |

- **Variation:** Fold the index fingers so that they touch the inside root of the thumbs. Straighten the other three fingers of each hand so that they are relaxed and slightly apart. Place the hand on the knees with palms facing downwards. Relax the hands and arms.

- ***Chin Mudra*** is performed the same way as 'Jnana Mudra,' except that the palms of both hands face upwards, with the backs of the hands resting on knees. Relax the hands and arms.

I have deliberately introduced you to the subject of 'Mudra' with the sub-subject of *'Hasta-Mudra.'* *'Mudra'* otherwise is a vast and complex subject in 'Yogic Sciences.' While on the topic, let me give some more fodder for *your academic interests* only.

'Mudra' a Sanskrit word means 'gesture' or 'attitude.' It may be defined as 'psychic, emotional, devotional and aesthetic gestures or attitudes.' Experts explain 'mudras' as attitude of energy flow, intended to link individual 'pranic' force (physical form) with universal or cosmic force. 'Mudra' also traces its root to the words *'mud'* (meaning 'delight' or 'pleasure') and *'dravay or dru'* (meaning 'to draw forth').

'Mudra' may also be understood as some kinds of 'seals,' 'short-cuts' or 'circuit-by-passes' introduced in bodily functions. These are combinations of subtle physical movements, having effects of altering mood, attitude, perceptions, awareness and concentration. Mudra may involve the whole body, or it may be a simple hand position.

Mudras manipulate the body's internal energies the same way that energy in the forms of sound and light gets diverted by a cliff face or a mirror. The internal energies which normally escape from the body and get dissipated into external words, get redirected within, by creating barriers within the body through mudra.

Mudras provide a means to access and influence the unconscious reflexes and primal, instinctive habit patterns that originate in the primitive areas of the brain around the brain stem. They establish a subtle, non-intellectual connection with these areas. Each mudra sets up a different link and has a correspondingly different effect on the body, mind and prana. The aim is to create fixed, repetitive postures and gestures which can snap the practitioner out of instinctive habit patterns and establish a more refined consciousness.

Thus, there are three groups of Yoga Mudras, Hasta-Mudra (Hand gestures), Mana-Mudra (Head gestures), and Kaya-Mudra (Body postural gestures). With this academic background let us come back to the topic of 'Hasta-Mudra.'

The sub-subject of Hand formations ('Hasta-Mudra') in Yogic Sciences is also quite vast. The scholars believe these formations to have a great influence on your body, heart and mind. The five fingers of our hands are believed to represent five elements: Agni (Fire)—Thumb, Vayu (Air) Forefinger or Index Finger, Akash (Sky)—Middle Finger, Prithvi (Earth) —Ring Finger and Jal (Water)—Little Finger. These postures are believed to have powers to cure many ailments. You may or may not find it easy to believe.

These claims are substantiated by a few of the curative sciences, particularly, those associated with Acupressure and Acupuncture. If interested, you may pick up a good book for advanced learning on these subjects.

The meditative hand mudras, very few of these being described here, redirect the energy/signal being emitted by the hands back into the body. Mudras which involve joining the thumb and index finger, engage the motor cortex at a very subtle level, generating a loop of energy which moves from the brain down the hand and then back again. Conscious awareness of this process rapidly leads to internalisation, thus facilitating meditation.

To facilitate your further learning, you are advised to practise and perfect the 'Salutation' (Namaskar) and 'Knowledge' (Jnana or Chin) formations. These two shall be extensively used in Meditation and Pranayama exercises. Some of the hand formations, with associated benefits are illustrated below:

3. Some More Hand Formations: (HASTA-MUDRAS)

Vayu Mudra

Press the forefinger at the first joint near the nail with your thumb as shown in the adjoining figure. (See 6.04) This helps reduce abdominal gases, reduces impact of tumours, (kampan) shivering and beneficial in paralysis.

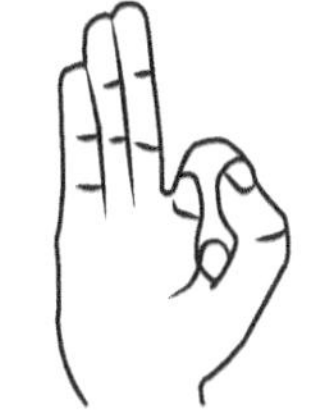

6.04: Vayu Mudra

Surya Mudra

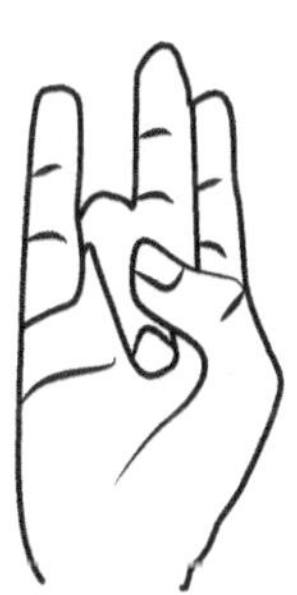

6.05: Surya Mudra

Press your thumb on the first joint of your ring finger as shown in figure. (See 6.05). This helps reduce obesity and excess weight. Both the thumb and ring finger carry a circuit connection like electricity because the veins of the ring finger are joined to the heart. It is believed in Hindu civilisation that by making a Tilak (apply vermilion on forehead) with the ring finger on someone's forehead, we transfer our strength to that person. That is the reason when the warriors went for war, a Tilak was applied by the mother or wife, for mental fortitude and strength.

Linga Mudra

Interlock the fingers of both hands as shown in figure 6.06. It helps cure cold, cough and throat problems.

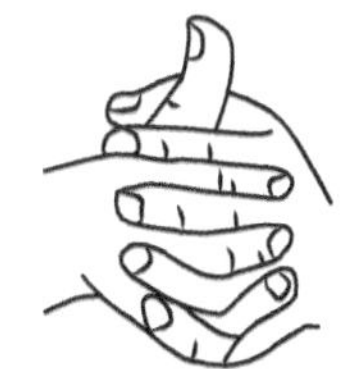

6.06: Linga Mudra

Prithvi Mudra

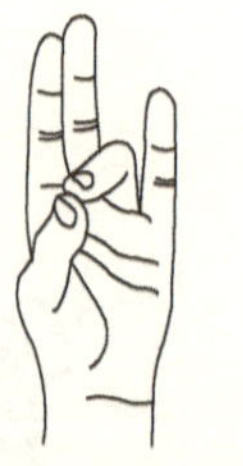

6.07: Prithvi Mudra

Performed by joining the ring finger and tip of the thumb, as shown in figure 6.07. Beneficial for thin skinny people, also brings radiance on the face. It is believed that the Prithvi mudra opens new horizons and transforms a narrow mind into a broader mind.

Shunya Mudra

Performed by pressing the middle finger at the joint by the thumb and holding it there exerting mild pressure as shown in figure 6.08. This mudra is beneficial for improving hearing powers.

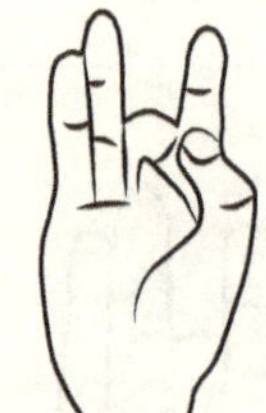

6.08: Shunya Mudra

Varun Mudra

This requires touching the tip of the little finger to the thumb as shown in figure 6.09. This is beneficial when the body is dehydrated. It is also known to remove the impurities from the blood.

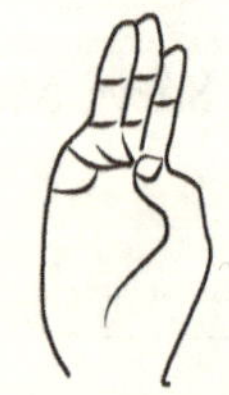

6.09: Varun Mudra

Hridaya Mudra

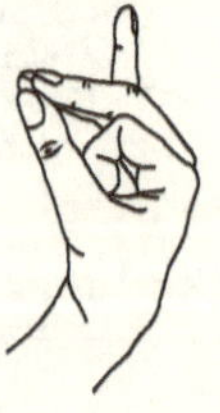

6.10: Hridya Mudra

Fold the index finger or forefinger and press it at the base of the thumb, except the little finger the middle two fingers should touch the thumb lightly as shown in figure 6.10. Beneficial for people with heart problems and people with a weak heart.

Practice for the Day

1. Observe how your routine postures were in your day-to-day activities, before reading this Chapter. See all the corrections that are required.

2. Practise the 'basic default posture' of 'spine/backbone straight,' and 'head high.'

3. Practise some of the hand formations. Particularly attain reasonable proficiency in perfecting the Namaskar and Jnana/Chin Mudra. These are essential for Meditation and Pranayama.

Tutorial for the Day

1. Ask some friend or colleague to take a few candid snap shots of you during the day, in your routine activities. Photographs/videos should cover some stairs climbing and descending activities, working on desks, using pen and paper/files, using Smartphone/Tablets, working on your Desktop/Laptop or other similar activities. Compare your postures with the ideal ones. If your workplace is having CCTV coverage, no need to bother anyone, just see footage of your recordings in the evening.

2. Practise Jnana Mudra, coupled with deep breathings, whenever you have some leisure time during the day sitting on your office chair/work-desk.

Day-Seven: The Yogic Postures: Part – II

Yogic Postures for Relaxation

Learning for the Day

Yogic Posture for Relaxation

Even if you may find it a bit repetitive, it is reiterated, that in all Yogic practices, relaxation is very important. After completion of one routine, one set of exercises, or on occurrence of laboured breathing, at the first hint of pain, overstretching of any limb, unbearable tension or stress on any muscle or sense of fatigue, whichever events occur first, you must change your posture to the nearest relaxation posture and relax there till you feel normal and ready to move on.

You should also not rush yourself into the next set of practice till your breathing becomes normal, your body feels good and your mind says "Hey man…! I am ready to conquer the world, tell me what I would do next for you!" Do not violate this golden rule. You will do more harm to yourself than good.

To logically and scientifically understand the utility and importance of relaxation in Yoga, you may like to understand the following concepts.

Some very sensitive internal organs perform the controls and regulatory functions. The control system is either open loop (See figure 7.01) or closed loop (See figure 7.02). These organs are generally called glands.

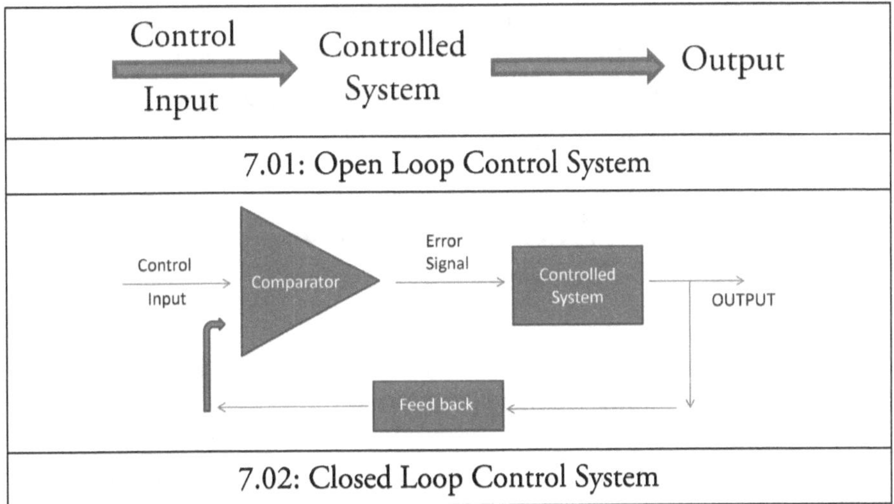

Such organs require a mere gesture, a prodding or a gentle reminder of their role, if dormant or not fully active. This gesturing/prodding/reminding is performed as part of the exercise routine. During relaxation phase these glands start performing properly their assigned role or may become hyperactive. The relaxation period must therefore be adequate to allow them just enough time to perform their role and return to normal state. During this phase they check, control, regulate and again go into hibernation.

On the other hand, the joints, bones, muscles, nerves and some oiling and lubricating systems respond to the Stretch-Hold-Release-Relax routines. During the relaxation phase the increase in suppleness and flexibility of joints, strengthening and toning of muscles and nerves and oiling and lubricating activities take place.

In order to overemphasize the utility of relaxation, I am deliberately teaching you first these relaxation postures. Yoga Asanas are performed in many starting postures, each posture having many of the Asanas. There is also a relaxation posture corresponding to each posture for Yoga Asanas. You are also expected to be in relaxed state before starting a fresh set of routine. So, these postures are your start point for that set of exercises. You may use any of the hand formations, while sitting in these postures,

Jnana Mudra being the default option. The starting postures are also referred to as 'Base position.' In Sanskrit 'Prarambh' means to start and 'Sthithi' means position. Thus, the starting postures (Asana) are also called as 'Prarambhic-sthithi' in Sanskrit and also in Hindi.

Practice for the Day:
The relaxation Postures:

Posture Number R1: Lyingd down Flat on Your Back: Corpse Posture (SHAVA-ASANA) (Supine Posture) (शवासन)

This is the important relaxation posture for all practices. So, it needs to be understood more carefully. This is also the 'default option' for all relaxation routines. Have you ever noticed the peace of a dead body? No stress, no facial expressions, no desires, no needs, no compulsion of false and unfelt greetings, no false smiles, no frowns, just peace, peace and more peace. Can we momentarily experience this pleasure, this feeling, while still living, surviving and thriving?

Steps:

1. Follow the prerequisites. Remember, early in the morning, neat clean environment, loose cotton clothes, outdoor or indoor, ground covered with a reasonably thick mat or blanket, with bed sheet on top, your mind, body, heart and soul all comfortable, at peace and in your control.

2. Lie down on your back; keep your body and all organs loose, the weight of your body being uniformly transferred to the ground. Let there be about one foot (300 millimetres) gap between your legs, your toes pointing towards the sky and heels resting comfortably on ground.

3. Your hands should be by the sides of your body, about one foot away from centre, thumbs and fingers loose, slightly bent inward and fingers pointing outward. Palm should be half open and

half closed. Head may be in centre or slightly tilted towards left or right, as comfortable.

4. Place the tongue pressed downwards and tip of tongue touching the lower gum line.

5. **Breathe** normally through the mouth using the air passage above the tongue, i.e., during inhalation, air should travel towards lungs using hollow space above tongue; similarly, during exhalation also air should take the same path.

6. Focus mind on focal point and consciously ask and nudge your brain and heart to relax, relax and relax. Keep counting the breaths.

7. **For deeper relaxation:** Consciously observe all your body parts for any sign of stress, pain, pressure, or over stretching from head to toe and toe to head. You may, if comfortable with it, say some prayers in your mind or do some chanting for relaxation or chant some mantra.

8. Lie down in this position, till your breathing is normal, till your body feels completely at ease.

9. This posture is also the starting posture (Base position) generally for all exercises to be performed lying down on back (Supine posture).

10. **Before proceeding for Exercises:** Tilt your complete body on one side, either right or left, get up slowly, taking supports of both hands, in lifting your body weight up.

7.03: Posture Number R1: Corpse Posture: Shavasana	7.04: Posture Number R2: Reversed Corpse Posture

Posture Number R2: Lying down Flat on the Stomach: The Reversed Corpse Posture (Prone Posture)

Steps:

1. Lie on the stomach. Stretch both arms above the head with the palms facing downward. The forehead should be resting on the floor. Relax the whole body in the same way as described for 'Shavasana' (Posture Number R1). If there is difficulty in breathing or a sense of suffocation is experienced, a pillow may be placed under the chest.

2. **Breathing:** Natural and rhythmic. The number of breaths may be counted as in 'Shavasana' while gently pushing the abdomen against the floor. For relaxation in the treatment of ailments, it should be performed for as long as possible. Before or during an asana session, a few minutes is sufficient.

3. **Focus:** Physical. On the breath, keep counting the number of breaths and relaxing the whole body.

4. For 'deeper relaxation' and 'before proceeding for exercise' same instructions as for 'Shavasana' apply.

Posture Number R3: The Comfortable Sitting Posture (Base Position) (PRARAMBHICSTITHI)

Steps:

1. Follow the prerequisites. Sit comfortably with your legs spread outwards in front, keeping about one foot (12 inches, 300 millimetres) gap between the two legs.

2. Take both your hands backwards, keeping palms and fingers well spread, pointing away from body, just a few centimetres behind the hips, providing support to upper part of body. Upper body weight should be equally balanced on both hands. The spine

should make an obtuse angle (Say about 100º) with surface plane.

3. Tilt your neck smoothly, slightly backward taking back side of your head as close to back(spine) as feasible, without overstretching. Open your mouth; place the tongue, pressed downwards, behind the lower jaw line. Fold tip of tongue backwards and touch the lower gum line. Breathe through the mouth normally. Stay in this position till you feel comfortable and ready to start the next routine/round of exercises. This is the relaxation posture as well as starting posture (Base position) for all exercises to be performed in sitting postures.

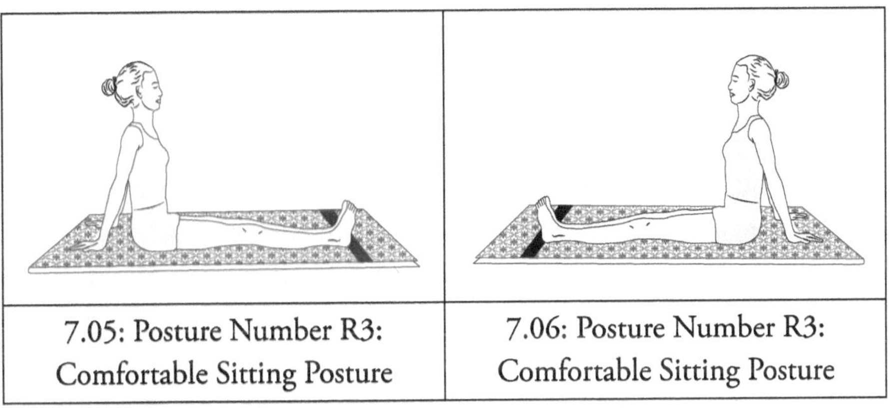

7.05: Posture Number R3: Comfortable Sitting Posture	7.06: Posture Number R3: Comfortable Sitting Posture

Posture Number R4: Lying down on Your Belly: The Crocodile Pose: MAKRA-ASANA (Prone Posture)

Precautions:

Persons suffering from lower back pains, back conditions and spinal problems should exercise due precautions.

Steps:

1. Lie down flat on your stomach. Weight of your body should be transferring to ground through as many pressure points as possible, legs and thighs resting on ground, transferring weight

of lower part of body to ground. Toe and leg fingers may be pointing downwards or slightly outwards, or inwards, as is felt more comfortable. Your stomach should be supporting weight of upper part of body. Chest should also be resting comfortably on ground.

2. Raise hands slightly upwards over your head. Now bend your right hand slightly, elbow pointing outwards, palm facing downwards. Place your palm beneath your forehead. Now take your left hand palm also and place it over your right hand palm, back side of palm facing upwards. Rest your head comfortably over these hand formations, with forehead firmly resting on back side of left hand palm.

3. Breathe normally. Rest in this position till breathing becomes normal and body comfortable.

4. You may also try variations. After placing right hand below forehead, palm facing upwards, tightly close the fist of left hand and place it over the back of right palm. Allow the focal point of your senses to rest on the cusp formed between the finger joints of first and second finger. Allow the weight of your head to be transferred to ground through the focal point, and the first cusp of left hand fist. Relax, enjoy and feel good.

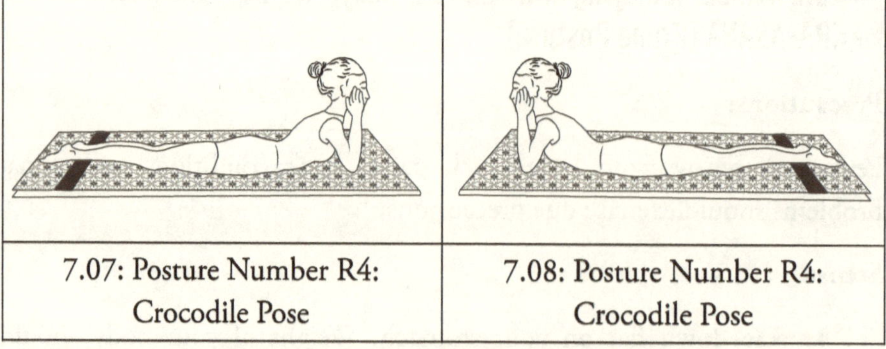

7.07: Posture Number R4: Crocodile Pose	7.08: Posture Number R4: Crocodile Pose

There are a few other positions for relaxation while lying on your belly. These are illustrated in pictures below.

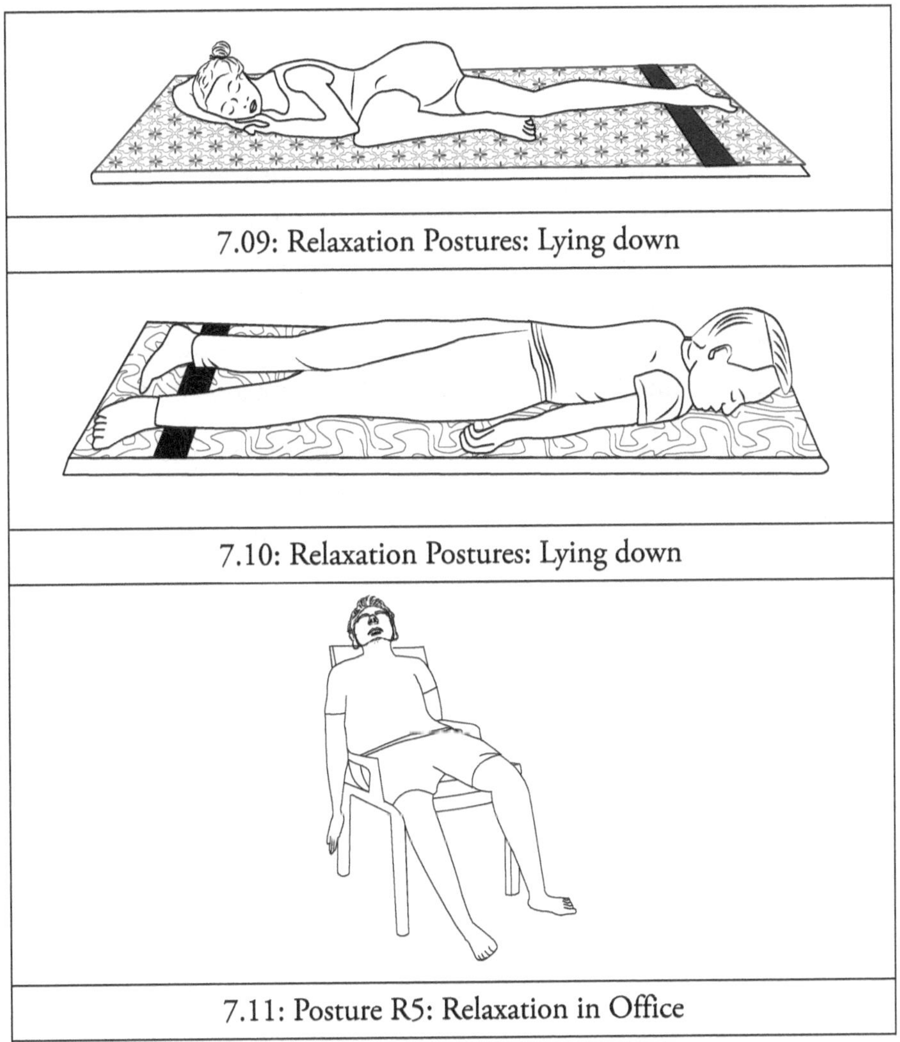

7.09: Relaxation Postures: Lying down

7.10: Relaxation Postures: Lying down

7.11: Posture R5: Relaxation in Office

Posture Number R5: Sitting on Chair: Relaxation in Office

You may comfortably relax, and refresh your body and mind, while still sitting on the office chair, by simply following the Yogic procedures of relaxing on chair. Next time when your feel physically tired or mentally exhausted, stressed and unable to focus and continue the office work, just take a five to ten minutes break and follow the steps detailed below.

Steps:

1. Place your body on the chair in corpse posture. Close the eyes. Allow arms to hang loosely by the side of the arm rests of the chair. Keep your mouth slightly open breathing normally in unforced manner through the mouth. Try and focus your attention on focal point or any other one single object/activity, not connected with routine office work. Mentally, slowly or if circumstances permit, loudly chant 'Aum' three times. (Refer Chapter-Two Day-Twelve).

2. After five to ten minutes when you open your eyes you will feel refreshed and ready to continue the mundane, monotonous, boring office work, with renewed vigour and enthusiasm.

Day-Eight: The Yogic Postures: Part – III

Yogic Postures Suitable for Meditation and Pranayama

Learning for the Day

In this section, we will learn some Yogic postures suitable for Meditation and Pranayama. Yogic postures as you know may be defined as 'comfortable positioning of body in some specific posture and holding it.' Your body needs to be in a relaxed and comfortable state, to enable mind to focus and relax in meditations and facilitate regulation of breathings during Pranayama.

Practice for the Day

Posture Number M1: Sitting Cross-Legged: Position of Happiness/Comfort. (SUKHA-ASANA)

This is the most important and easiest posture for all Meditation and Pranayama exercises. Persons unable to sit in the more difficult meditation postures can utilise this posture without any adverse effects. This posture facilitates attainment of mental and physical balances, without stresses, strains and pains.

Steps:

1. Follow the prerequisites.

2. Sit comfortably with your legs spread outwards in front, keeping about one foot (12 inches, 300 millimetres) gap between the two legs. Keep your hands either by the sides of hips or behind

your hips, as comfortable, to maintain balance. Keep the body fully relaxed by keeping upper body tilted slightly backwards and taking support of hands for transferring the weight of the upper body to the ground. (Base position, Posture Number R3).

3. Take your hands off the floor, and push your upper body slightly in front, such that your backbone, slightly stretched upwards, acquires a vertical position. The backbone and neckline, with head held high, should be perpendicular to the ground.

4. Now catch hold of your right leg, by supporting and nudging the right foot with your right hand or both hands so that the right heel reaches the point on the floor just beneath the reproductive organ. Place the right foot under the left thigh touching the surface, with heel touching the parting line of buttocks, at bottommost point, or as near as feasible, taking adequate care to place the reproductive organ carefully away from heel.

5. Catch hold of your left leg also, by supporting and nudging the foot with hands, place the left foot under the right thigh. The two lines connecting the heel and toe in both your feet make a "V" formation. See pictures 8.01 below.

6. Rest your relaxed palms on the knees in 'jnana' or 'chin' mudra. Hands should be loosely hanging for relaxation and meditation. For Pranayama, you may slightly stretch your hands. Keep the head, neck and back loose, un-stretched, tension-free but straight and upright.

7. **Breathing:** Normal, meditatively slow and unforced.

8. **Focus: Mind:** To concentrate on focal point. Consciousness of time and mental counting of breaths/exercise to be followed. Eyes: Closed and shut for Meditation and Pranayama exercises. Ears: Enjoying the peace of silence or pleasures of soft music.

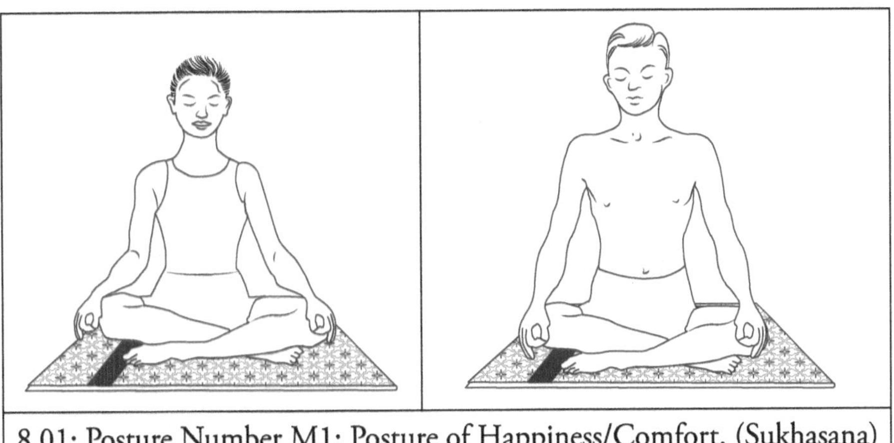

8.01: Posture Number M1: Posture of Happiness/Comfort. (Sukhasana)

'Sukhasana' is a relaxation posture to be used after extended periods of sitting in the more difficult posture of 'Padmasana' (Posture M3) or 'Siddhasana' (Posture M4). It looks simple, but is difficult to sustain for longer durations unless knees are close to or touching the ground. Buttocks bearing the burden of body weight may develop mild backache. Other postures provide larger contact area between lower parts of body and ground and smoother weight transfer. These postures are therefore suitable for longer duration of meditation.

Posture Number M2: Sitting Cross-Legged: Half Lotus Posture. (ARDH-PADMA-ASANA)

This is also an important posture for all Meditation and Pranayama exercises, next to 'Sukhasana' in difficulty level. Persons suffering from sciatica or sacral-disorders should refrain from performing this posture.

Steps:

1. Attain posture as in 'Sukhasana' (Posture Number M1)

2. Now place your left foot on the right thigh, as close to or as ahead of thigh as possible without overstretching. This is the Half Lotus posture ('Ardhpadmasana').

3. You may also practise it with legs placed the other way around, i.e., right foot on left thigh. During practising the posture or performing meditation or some Pranayama exercise sitting in this posture, position of legs may be changed from left to right, if pain or pressure is felt in leg or on thigh.

4. **Breathing:** Generally normal, meditatively slow and unforced.

5. **Focus: Mind:** To concentrate on focal point, consciousness of time and mental counting of breaths/exercise to be followed. Eyes: Closed and shut for Meditation and Pranayama exercises. During performance of some exercise sitting in this posture, eyes may remain closed or open and closely observing and guiding organs for that specific exercise, the way the exercise is prescribed.

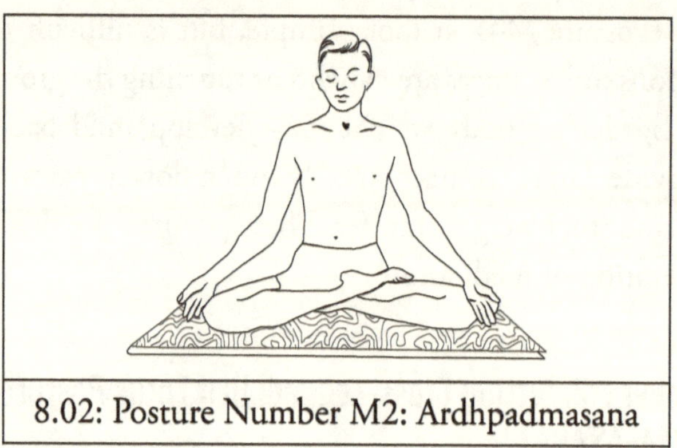

8.02: Posture Number M2: Ardhpadmasana

Posture Number M3: Sitting Cross-Legged: Lotus Posture. (PADMA-ASANA)

This is the most important posture for all Meditation and Pranayama exercises. Amongst the various poses prescribed for meditation, Padmasana is unique and foremost. It holds the most conspicuous place in all the Yoga practices.

It is called Padmasana because of its full pose lending one the appearance of a full-blown lotus. Persons suffering from sciatica, sacral infections, and with weak, injured or post-surgery knees should not perform this. This posture is difficult with stiff bones and joints. It is advisable to develop some flexibility of knees by other subtle exercises (Refer Chapter-Three), and meditation postures before attempting this.

Steps:

1. Sit in the Sukhasana (Posture Number M1). Stretch the legs forward, place the right foot gently on left thigh, at the left hip joint, and the left foot similarly at the right thigh, at right hip joint.

2. The soles should face upwards and the heels should be close to the pubic zone. Keep the spine erect. Place the right hand on the right knee joint and the left hand on the left knee joint. Palms formed in 'Jnana' or 'chin' mudra. Close the eyes focussing on focal point or gaze gently at the tip of the nose. Keep body relaxed.

3. Relax the arms with the elbows slightly bent and check that shoulders are not raised, hunched or drooping. This is Padmasana. Practise this Asana for five minutes to start with and gradually increase the time to one to two hours. When sitting in one posture feels difficult, bend the other leg and place the foot on top of the opposite thigh. Both knees should ideally touch the ground in the final position.

4. Be attentive towards the total posture of the body. Make necessary adjustments by moving forward or backward till comfortable alignment and uniformity in weight transfer is attained. Perfect alignment and good contact area for weight transfer are key to correct posture of Padmasana.

5. Padmasana is said to destroy all diseases and bestows quick emancipation to the practitioner. Breathing and focus shall remain same as for above postures.

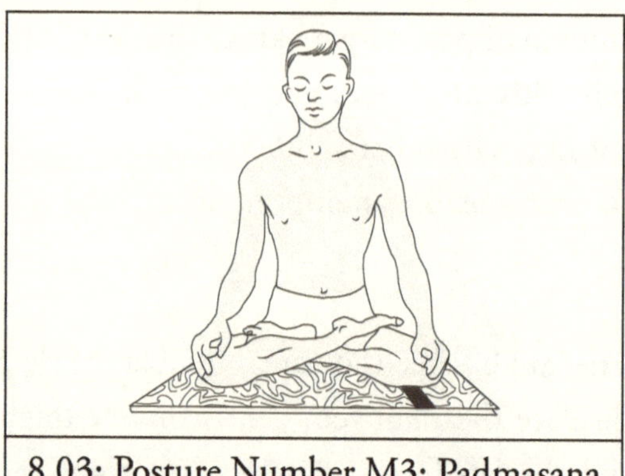

8.03: Posture Number M3: Padmasana

Calmness and steadiness of body are prime requirements for meditation. 'Padmasana' allows the body to be held completely steady and firm for longer durations. Your body attains structural stability, with legs formation acting as firm foundation, trunk and spine acting like a column (pillar) supporting and keeping the head (mind, brain) steady, firm and ready to face winds, storms and earthquakes of stresses and emotional turbulences.

The pressure on the lower spine has a relaxing effect on the nervous system. With the slow breathings and decreased muscular tensions, the blood pressure gets reduced. In normal state large blood flows are directed towards the legs, keeping in view the needs of the tough tasks handled of providing mobility. During Padmasana this blood flow gets directed towards the abdominal region. The coccygeal and sacral nerves get toned up and digestion process gets stimulated.

Posture Number M4: The Accomplished Pose for Men. (SIDDHA-ASANA)

Precautions:

This posture should not be practised by those with sciatica or sacral infections. Take extreme care not to cause injury to the male reproduction organs. This is a moderately difficult posture like Padmasana.

Steps:

1. Sit with the legs straight in front of the body, in the same manner as prior to starting practice for Sukhasana (Posture Number M1). Bend the right leg and place the sole of the foot flat against the inner left thigh with the heel pressing the perineum (the area midway between the genitals and the anus), sitting on top of the right heel. This is an important aspect of Siddhasana.

2. Adjust the body until it is comfortable, and the pressure of the heel is firmly applied. Bend the left leg and place the left ankle directly over the right ankle so that the ankle bones are touching, and the heels are one above the other.

3. Press the pubis with the left heel directly above the genitals. The genitals will, therefore, lie between the two heels.

4. If this last position is too difficult, simply place the left heel as near as possible to the pubis. Push the toes and the outer edge of the left foot into the space between the right calf and thigh muscles. If necessary, this space may be enlarged slightly by using the hands or temporarily adjusting the position of the right leg. Grasp the right toes and pull them up into the space between the left calf and thigh. Again, adjust the body so that it is comfortable.

5. The legs should now be locked, with the knees touching the ground and the left heel directly above the right heel. Make the spine erect and feel as though the body is fixed on the floor. Place the hands on the knees in 'jnana,' or 'chin' mudra. Close the eyes and relax the whole body. There is a feminine version of this Asana too.

Only a few of the meditation postures to enable you to start practising meditation are being described here. Once you attain some proficiency and perfection in these postures, explore for more. In particular, gather information about 'Siddha-Yoni-Asana' (for girls), 'Swastikasana,' 'Dhayanveerasana' and 'Simhasana.' In case meditation is your prime motivator for adoption of Yoga in life, perfect these postures to the minutest details. For the common practitioner reasonable perfections in Sukhasana, and Ardhpadmasana, are sufficient to start the subtle physical exercises and earn the benefits of Yoga.

Day-Nine: The Yogic Postures: Part – IV

The Starting Postures (Base Positions)

Learning for the Day

In this section, we will learn some Yogic postures, which are the starting postures (Base positions) for the subtle exercises (Sukshma-Vyayama) or Yogic exercises (Yoga Asana). These postures are also invariably the resting positions (relaxation postures) for exercises. There are some deliberate repetitions here, to facilitate sequential learnings in each series.

Posture Number S1: Sitting, Legs in Front, Hands Back

This is the easiest posture. This is the starting posture (Base position) for many subtle exercises (Sukshma – Vyayama) and Yoga Asanas, which are performed in sitting positions with legs remaining in front stretched outwards, away from body and parallel to each other. You have already learnt this posture as Posture Number R3 ('Prarambhic-sthithi'). It is being repeated here for the sake of continuity and ease of understanding.

Steps:

1. Sit comfortably with your legs spread outwards in front, keeping about one foot (12 inches, 300 millimetres) gap between the two legs.

2. Take both your hands backwards, keeping palms and fingers well spread, pointing away from body, providing support to the upper part of body. Upper body weight should be equally balanced on

both hands. The spine should make an obtuse angle (say about 100°) with the surface plane.

3. **For relaxation:** Tilt your neck smoothly slightly backwards taking back side of your head as close to back(spine) as feasible, without overstretching. Open your mouth; place the tongue behind the lower jaw line. Breathe through the mouth normally. Stay in this position till you feel comfortable and ready to start the next routine/round of exercises.

4. **Before proceeding for Exercises:** Join both legs together. Push your head smoothly in front to make head in line with spine. Push the upper portion of body, with supports of your hands to make spine in vertical position to the surface plane. Release and free both hands. Point your toes. Focus attention and eyes as per demand of exercises. Take a deep breath. You are ready.

Posture Number S2: Sitting Legs Backwards, below the Buttocks (VAJRA-ASANA)

This also is an important posture for all meditation, Pranayama and Sukshma-Vyayama exercises next to 'Sukhasana.' There is a series of Yoga Asana for which Vajrasana is the starting and relaxing position. This posture is also very beneficial for the complete digestion system. It offers suppleness to ankles, shanks, calves, hamstrings and knees. With stiff joints and bones there may be some difficulties initially in attaining perfections in this posture.

Unlike other Yogic practices, wherein empty bowels and belly is one of the standard prerequisites, this Asana can be performed after meals. If fact, if you develop the habit of sitting in this Asana for five to fifteen minutes after every meal every day, you will never suffer from any indigestion related ailments, i.e., acidity, acute indigestion, constipation and gastric conditions, etc. It is a perfect Yogic substitute for all laxatives.

Precaution:

Avoid doing this if there is severe pain in the knees.

Steps:

1.   Sit on the floor with the legs extended.

2.   Fold one leg at knee, by nudging and supporting it with hands and smoothly rotating it outwards in a semi-circular manner and keep the foot under the bottom, with either heel or toe touching the parting line of hips.

3.   With the support of hands, shift the body weight carefully on the folded leg.

4.   Then fold the other leg in the same manner and place the other heel or toe also below the buttocks, with either heel or toe placed beneath the parting line of buttocks. Readjust the body weight uniformly on both buttocks. Knees may be kept together.

5.   Keep the spine straight. Close the eyes and sit stable. Ensure smooth transfer of body weight from upper portion to feet placed below buttocks, and through feet to the ground. Place the hands on the knees, in Jnana mudra, palms down. Breathe normally through nostrils. Focus attention on the flow of air passing through nostrils. This is one variation of the final posture of this Asana.

6.   You may also attain this final posture by kneeling on the floor, bringing the big toes together and separating the heels and lowering the buttocks onto the inside surface of the feet with the heels touching the sides of hips.

7.   Practise this Asana as frequently and for as long a duration as possible, especially directly after meals, for minimum five minutes

to enhance the functioning of the digestion system. If suffering from severe digestive disorders, sit in 'Vajrasana' and practise abdominal breathings for minimum hundred counts before and after meals.

8. Check the flow of breath through the nostrils. If the air flow through the left nostril is more prominent, place the left big toe on top of right big toe. If flow on right side is prominent, place the right toe on top. This will help in balancing the flow of breath in both nostrils.

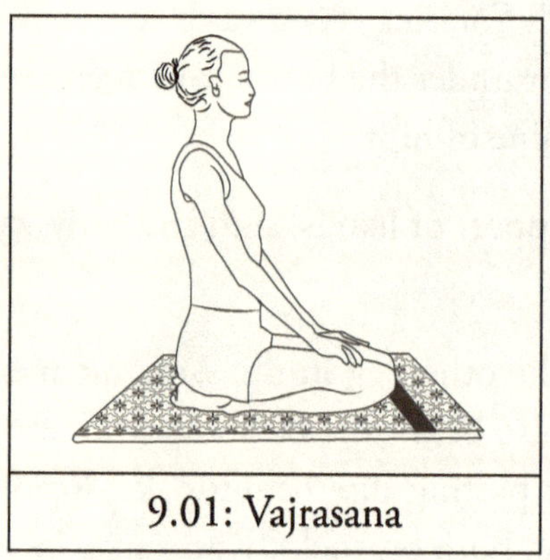

9.01: Vajrasana

9. **Variations:** This Asana can be performed in four different ways, depending upon the location and direction of feet placed below buttocks, the upper portion remaining the same in all four variations. These are illustrated below.

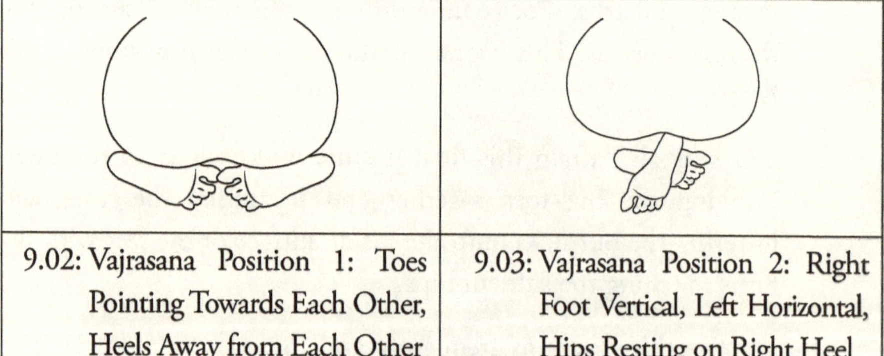

9.02: Vajrasana Position 1: Toes Pointing Towards Each Other, Heels Away from Each Other	9.03: Vajrasana Position 2: Right Foot Vertical, Left Horizontal, Hips Resting on Right Heel

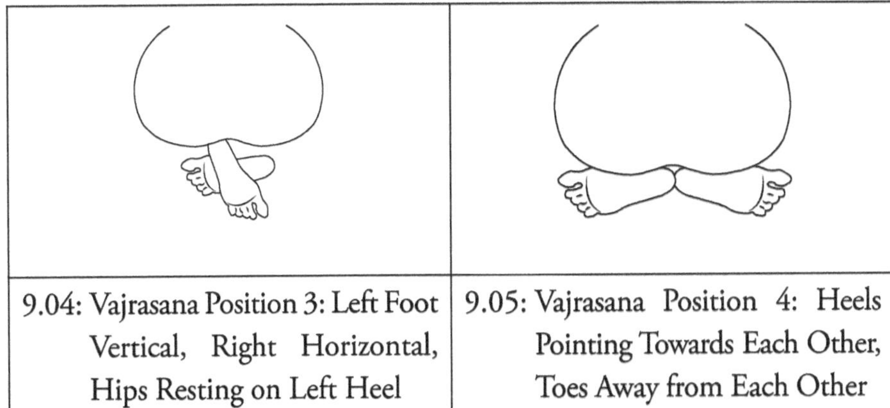

9.04: Vajrasana Position 3: Left Foot Vertical, Right Horizontal, Hips Resting on Left Heel	9.05: Vajrasana Position 4: Heels Pointing Towards Each Other, Toes Away from Each Other

'Vajra' (meaning 'thunderbolt') is believed to be the weapon of 'Indra' (believed in 'Hindu way of life' to be the 'King of gods,' just as mind is king of human body and all senses). The 'Vajra-Asana' series is very beneficial for reproduction and digestion systems. After you attain significant perfection in the basic posture, you may try some more difficult versions.

Version 1: Separate the feet, keeping knees together, so that the big toes are about twenty-five centimetres apart. Keep spine straight.

Version 2: Place a rolled-up towel or blanket on the floor between the legs. Separate the feet, keeping knees together, about twenty-five centimetres. Sit on the towel/blanket in 'Vajrasana.'

Posture Number S3: Standing Erect Like a Mountain (TADA-ASANA)

This Asana derives its name from mountain, as it involves standing tall, erect, rigid, proud and majestic like a mountain.

Steps:

1. Stand straight, erect, legs joined together as close to each other as feasible. The heels and big toes should touch each other.

2. Tighten the knee and pull the knee caps up, contracting the hips and pulling up the muscles at the back of the thighs.

3. Keep the stomach in, chest forward, spine straight and stretched upwards and neck straight. Head should be held high.

4. Uniformly balance the body weight equally on heels and toes.

5. Place arms by the side of thighs, parallel to the body, the fingers together and pointing downwards.

6. In Step 1 to 5 above, we have performed stretching the complete body upwards, in an apparent effort to gain some extra height and stature causing the sequential stretching action from bottom (knees) to top (neck). You may alternatively cause similar stretching action from top (neck) to bottom (knees).

7. This is the starting and warming up posture for all Asanas performed standing up. This is also the posture for relaxing when tired in exercises, in standing posture.

8. For relaxation, de-stretch the complete body sequentially, loosening all internal organs and external body parts, keep arms and palms loosely hung, breathe normally. Before proceeding for exercises, stretch up the body again.

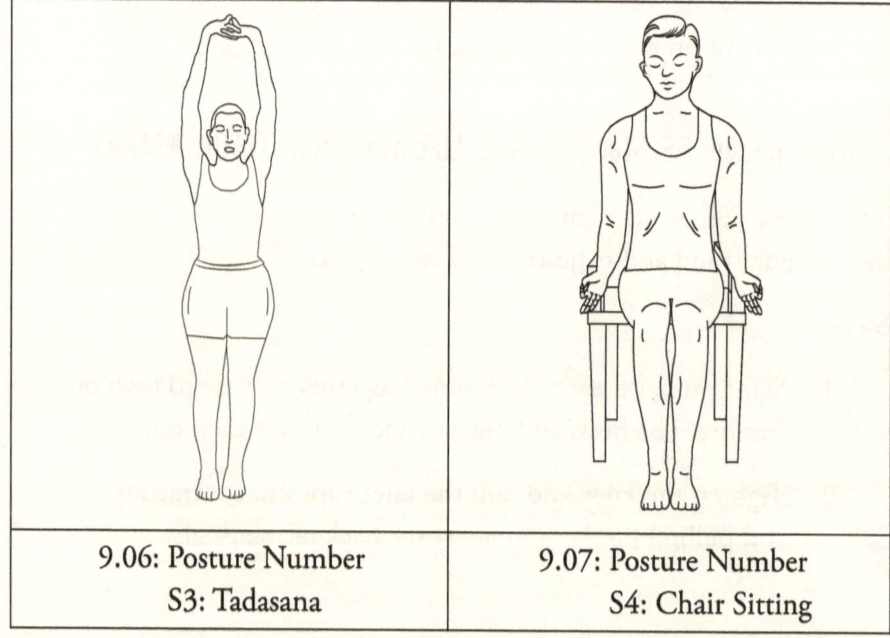

9.06: Posture Number S3: Tadasana	9.07: Posture Number S4: Chair Sitting

Posture Number S4: Sitting on Chair

Just in case you are suffering from some physical infirmities, are physically challenged, or suffering from severe back pains, and are unable to sit down or stand properly, you may still perform some of the Yoga routines, by sitting comfortably on chair. Take the following precautions.

1. Chair height should be adequate to enable you to sit comfortably with your legs bent at ninety degrees allowing your feet to comfortably rest on floor, lower part of legs between knee and heels remaining parallel to the legs of chair.

2. Armrests should be flexible or cushioned, allowing you to rest and support your arms on armrests for longer durations.

3. There must be no protruding nails or unnecessary projections of wood or any other material obstructing movements of hands and legs. You should be able to take up and down and rotate your arm freely making your shoulder as hinge.

4. Edges of armrests must be smooth or cushioned. If not, it makes sense to wrap two towels one on each armrest, so that you may comfortably place your hands on edges and corners of armrests.

5. **For relaxation:** Sit comfortably, legs bent at knees at ninety degrees angle, heels, feet and toes resting on floor. Hands should be dropping down from shoulder, arms comfortable resting on full length of armrest, spine straight, and head tilted slightly backwards, mouth slightly open. Breath normally though mouth.

6. You may perform meditation, Pranayama and Sukshama-Vyayama, involving legs, arms, neck, upper torso, etc., sitting on chair.

Summary of Postures

The summary of postures learnt so far, is presented in tabular manner as under:-

Table of the Day

Before attaining starting posture	Starting posture	General posture during exercises	Type of exercises	Relaxation posture
Follow prerequisites	S1	M1 or M2 or M3 or M4	Meditation, Pranayama	R1 or R2 or R3 or R4
R3	S1	S1	Subtle exercises, sitting postures	R3 or R1
R1	R1	As per instruction of the exercise	Subtle exercises or Yogasana—lying down on back posture (Supine posture)	R1
R2	R2 or R4	As per instruction of the exercise	Subtle exercises or Yogasana—lying down on stomach posture (Prone posture)	R2 or R4
S3 (Relaxed)	S3 (Body stretched)	S3 (Body stretched)	Subtle exercises or Yogasana—standing posture	S3 (Relaxed)

Exercise for the Day

1. Practise 'Padmasana,' 'Tadasana,' and 'Vajrasana' (all four variants). Attaining reasonable proficiency and perfections in postures in 'Ardhpadmasana' and 'Sukhasana,' should not be a problem by now.

2. Remember to perform 'Shavasana,' for minimum five minutes before closing your practice.

Tutorial for the Day

1. There are many other postures, much more complex and intricate than those described here. If interested in higher levels of learning, find out more about these from various sources.

Day-Ten: Your Weekend Detoxification (Detox) Package

Learning of the Day

Now that you have learnt the basics and are familiar with the difficult sounding names of 'Sukhasana,' 'Padmasana,' 'Vajrasana,' you can also comfortably achieve some semblance to pictures depicting these postures. You may be eager to start some real practise. However, I want some more preparations. You should migrate to the real practice sessions after some detoxification of body. So, here is my packaged weekend-detoxification-program for you.

Precautions first! You should try this only if you are in good health conditions. If you are suffering from any disease or ailments, do not try this, except under medical supervision and expert's advice. If you are suffering from any discomfort associated with the digestion system, do not even think of attempting this. Also, if there is some pain in lower limbs, foot, legs, knees or thighs, do not attempt sitting in 'Vajrasana.'

I am assuming for this section that you enjoy two days for weekend. In case you are not the fortunate ones, I request you to try this, whenever you have an opportunity of being able to spare at least two relaxed days for this package.

Before starting, have light meals, at least two days prior to weekend, i.e., Thursday and Friday. All three meals, i.e., breakfast, lunch, and dinner should be light. It shall be best if you may squeeze in some extra fresh fruits and green vegetables in your meals. If you are fond of your evening snacks, they should also be light on your belly, non-fried, non-oily, less in carbohydrates and rich in fibres. Also drink lots of water. At least double the quantity of your normal water intake. Even otherwise, liquid intakes should be more than your normal routines. If you are a casual smoker or social drinker, remember—no smoking, no alcohol, at least two days before and after the weekend. Keep all toxins away for effective detoxification.

For This Package, You Will Need

1. Plenty of potable water.

2. Some additives/adulterants—to make your excessive drinking of water palatable. Suggestions are: Honey and fresh lime juice (Fresh lemons), Apple Cider Vinegar, Spiced Buttermilk, fresh fruit juices, aloe-vera or any other similar liquid to make water tasty and palatable to facilitate drinking in large quantities. In case you are comfortable with drinking pure unadulterated water, no additives are required. Additive should also not contain any additional sugar, artificial flavourings or preservatives.

3. Green tea—To bring some variation to fluids intakes.

4. Knowledge and perfections in postures for sitting in all four variants of 'Vajrasana,' (Refer Chapter-One – Day-Nine (Posture Number S2)) for long duration sittings (ten to twenty minutes) in one stretch.

5. Easy access to loo.

6. Gas Stove/Induction cook top/electric kettle or other device to heat up the water.

Steps:

1. Observe precautions as advised for at least two days prior to starting.

2. First thing in the morning, prepare one and half (1½) to two (2) litres of lukewarm water. Water should be at temperature

5 to 10 degree centigrade above room temperature only. It should be neither too hot, nor cold; just lukewarm.

3. Add one table spoon of honey. Stir gently so that honey gets dissolved. Add fresh juice of one medium size lemon (about one table spoon of lemon juice) to this lukewarm water.

4. Drink this water, two to three glasses at a time, as per capacity, giving two to five minutes (or longer, if required) of break in between each drinking sessions. You should do some brisk walking, jogging or similar light exercises during the break periods. You may also perform some light exercises involving up, down and sideways movements of hands, light jumping, skipping, cycling or anything that suits your fancy. Urinate as frequently as required.

5. Immediately after finishing drinking the full quantity, sit in Vajrasana for ten to fifteen minutes. You may keep on changing the foot positions for giving relief to foot. Try out all four variants of Vajrasana. Keep on changing positions from Position 1 (Toes pointing towards each other, heels away from each other) to Position 2 (Right foot vertical, left horizontal, hips resting on right heel) and so on.

6. While sitting in Vajrasana, you are likely to experience some abdominal sounds, the growling and rumbling sounds in your belly. They are normal. Make no attempt to control or suppress them. Allow these to occur naturally.

7. Repeat steps No 1 to 5, at least three times during the day. For variations, instead of honey and lime, use Apple Cider Vinegar (in lukewarm water), buttermilk, fruit juice, etc. (water at room temperature). Drinking of 1 ½ to 2 litres of water followed by ten to fifteen minutes of Vajrasana is the key ingredient of this package.

8. Do not consume any heavy meals during the day. You may eat as much fruits as you like. Fruits of water melon, cantaloupe,

musk-melon, cucumber, honey dew, Galia melon, and papaya variety are best. If it is difficult to control the pangs of hunger, you may consume light meals like:

- Khichdi (rice and split pulses (lentils), cooked together by shallow frying in ghee (clarified butter) and boiling with light herbs and spices in plenty of water).

- Fresh vegetable soups.

- Split pulses (like Moong dal) cooked with plenty of water.

This is a good package for detoxification of your body. If you can perform six to seven rounds of these steps in the two weekend days, you will feel fresh and energised. You may also lose ½ to 2 kilograms weight.

If you are already health-conscious and had been following some other diet-control or detox measures, you are at liberty to follow your own routines. But it is an important preparation before starting actual Meditation and Pranayama sessions. Do not ignore my advice. Primary requirement of meditation is ability to control and regulate the brain. And primary consideration for effective Pranayama is ability to regulate breath. Both require the body to be reasonably clean and devoid of accumulated wastes and toxins. The focus of mind and control of breath become easier with a detoxed body.

This completes your learning about the heart and the core of Yoga. If you are ready, we will start learning meditation from tomorrow onwards.

Chapter-Two

Meditation

Day-Eleven: Chanting for Fun and Relaxation

Learning for the Day

I sincerely hope that you have gone through the prescribed detox procedure or some other similar procedure of fasting, fruit-diet, controlled-diet, etc. This is essential to smoothen your further learning. Learning ahead is going to be tough on your thought process.

You should by now have observed my repeated usage of the phrase **'Relax…! Relax…!! and… Relax!!!'**

This usage was deliberate, to lead you to this part of learning. Chanting and recitation of some distinct words or phrases holds great significance in meditation practices. Our rational and logical mind may show some resistance in accepting this.

We will learn how chanting of certain combination of sounds, words, phrases, sentences and 'mantras' is beneficial for our mind, emotions and body in later parts of this Chapter.

For the time being, let us Relax, by making the sounds of 'Reee…laaa…xxxx,' i.e., by loudly pronouncing the word by dragging all three sounds of 'RREE,' 'LLAA' and 'XX' a bit longer, then in normal pronunciation. How does it feel?

Now perform any exercise you are familiar with, to tire your body and to make your breathing laboured. Count the breathings, time spent and numbers of exercise routines. Once you are fatigued with forced breathings, go to nearest relaxation posture and relax. Count the breathings till breathing becomes normal.

Now repeat the above exercise with a variation. While relaxing chant 'Reee…laaa…xxxx' and 'Relax… Relax…and Relax!' loudly. How do you feel? Was it better? Did you achieve the normal breathing earlier? You may also repeat the same exercise with one more variation. While relaxing and chanting, consciously nudge your mind, heart, and tired body parts to relax.

Chanting works on various levels on you, positive-auto-suggestion being one of these. Pick up any book on modern management or self-improvement and you will find a few chapters dedicated to this subject. Yogic routines beautifully incorporate this concept in its package of practices. A specific specialized sub-subject also deals with talking to your body organs as a curative measure.

Now, if I have been able to convince you on positive effects of chanting, can you chant with me the following:

Relax my Body! Relax my Mind!
Relax my Heart! Relax my Soul!
Relax! Relax! and Relax!

Repeat the above chant while relaxing lying down in Shavasana after performing a tiresome set of exercises.

Now, let us add some elements of feelings and emotions to the physical and mechanical ways of producing sounds. Mentally try to talk to your body, mind, heart and soul to relax during above chanting. Nudge them, guide them, tell them "Everything is perfect," "I am at peace," "I am feeling better," "I am getting better," "All the ailments and disorders are disappearing from my body" or similar positive sentences. Chanting accompanied with positive mental activities does work better. Try it! Perform some physical exercises, get fatigued, and lie down in Shavasana, chanting the above phrases and sentences.

In the phases of relaxation, smaller ones between two routines, medium ones on tiring and the longer ones at the end of long practice sessions, it is strongly recommended that you chant, while relaxing. It will take significant time to feel the subtle differences that chanting makes. But believe me! Once you start feeling the difference, it is huge.

Practice for the Day

Practise the chanting of the following sentences, adding some music, rhythm, beats and emotions of your own liking. You may like to first attain a state of moderate tiredness by some physical exercises and try the chanting, while relaxing.

Buddham Sharnam Gacchami! (Hey Lord Buddha! here I come to you for shelter!) *Ananadam Sharnam Gacchami!* (I am going towards the shelter of Happiness.) *Yogam Sharnam Gacchami!* (Yoga! I seek shelter beneath you!) *Guruwar Sharnam Gacchami!* (Hey teacher! I seek knowledge from you!)	बुध्धम शरणम् गच्छामि। आनंदम शरणम् गच्छामि। गूरुवर शरणम् गच्छामि। योगम शरणम् गच्छामि।
My body is healthy! My heart is at peace! My mind is happy!	मेरा शरीर स्वस्थ है। मेरा हृदय शांत है। मेरा मन प्रसन्न है।
'Aum Shanti!' 'Aum Shanti!' 'Aum Shanti!' 'Shanti!' 'Shanti!' 'Shanti!'	ॐ शांति! ॐ शांति! ॐ शांति! शांति! शांति! शांति!

Tutorial for the Day

1. Create a few relaxation chants of your own, for your own use, in your own mother tongue or the language you are most comfortable with. Make it a bit musical and rhythmic, so that there are ample variations in sounds, resulting into good variations in vibrations of your vocal chords. They should carry some positive thought for the universe, nature, humanity or yourself.

2. Now that you know the importance of chanting in the light of positive-auto-suggestions, can you ponder and analyse the positives and negatives of the environment around you? The sources of entertainment, the television, movies, news in electronic, print and social media, etc. Are they positive or negative? Are they serving you violence, rape and murder stories, revenge, tragedies, tear-jerkers, or making some attempt to make you feel relaxed, make you happy, smile and laugh? Can you do something to make your surroundings a bit more positive? Can you at least insulate yourself from all the negativities surrounding you? Food for thought! A small change from negativities to positives may change your life.

3. It may also do lots of good to you, if you closely observe the colours surrounding you, in your bedroom, drawing room and most importantly around the place chosen for your Yogic routines. Keeping in mind the hypothesis that sharp and darker colours like red carry some associations to violence, colours like dark black to gloom, and colours like green and white are universally associated with peace. Choose the colours around you according to your desirable emotions. Also, do not forget to make the place chosen for Yoga a bit more fragrant and green or white. If you are not convinced on my hypothesis on colours, ask an electrical engineer, why all electrical machines are primarily painted in grey colours.

Day-Twelve: Ohm ('AUM') Chanting and Recitations

Learning for the Day

'Aum' or **'Ohm'** (ॐ) is considered the most sacred sound in 'Hinduism,' as well as a few other religions originated in the Indian continent, i.e., 'Buddhism,' 'Jainism,' and 'Sikhism.' It is a spiritual icon in 'Hindu's way of life.' It is one of the most sacred symbols in 'Hinduism.' Hindus believe 'Aum' to be the universal name of the creator, the Supreme Being, and that it surrounds all of creation. The "Amen" in Christianity and "Ameen" for Muslims also shows a common linguistic ancestry. It is believed to symbolise the personality of God. It symbolises life breath. It is the most chanted sound symbol. It is believed to have the most profound effect on the body, mind and soul of the chanter.

I fully understand that the above explanation of the importance of the sound of a sacred symbol may be offensive to your sensibilities. This elaboration would not be in harmony with your thoughts. When there is no creator, how can there be a sound of creation? How can creator have a personality? And what am I trying to do here? Lead you on the path of Hinduism, spirituality, a human God, (that too, a narcissist who blesses you on hearing his favourite sounds)? Am I trying to make you believe in 'Nirwana' (Detachment), 'Moksha' (Salvation) and Rebirth? No! My dear friends, these are none of my intentions. So, here goes my own alternative explanation of the importance of the sound, the importance of chanting 'Aum' or 'Ohm.'

Ohm (Symbol: Ω) is the unit of measurement of electrical resistance, named after the German physicist Georg Simon Ohm. Electrical resistance is the resistance (akin to friction in movements) exhibited by an electrical conductor, towards flow of current. A bit of scientific explanations here will cause no harm.

Electrical current flows between two points at different electrical potential, when joined together by a conductor (one that has less electrical resistance, normally metals like silver, aluminium and copper). Electrical potential is a measure of availability of electrical charge, i.e., presence of agitated and ready to move free electrons, carrying negative charge on their body.

The point having larger presence of free electrons is at negative charge. The one receptive to electrons is at positive charge. Just as water flows from higher to lower levels, electrical current flows from positive to negative. So does heat from high to low temperatures. Everything in nature flows from higher to lower. And this fellow, electrical resistance tries to stop this flow of current like a villain.

Now, Ohm the inventor of resistance was a great narcissist. He left a legacy behind him. He wants you to chant his name. He will reduce or remove his creation, i.e., the resistance to the flow of knowledge to you, and the flow of good health and happiness towards you. Are you convinced with my twisted logic? No? Okay! Do you appreciate my efforts in convincing you? Yes! Okay! Will you please chant a loud 'Aum' for my satisfaction?

Now that I have made my intentions clear, I want you to believe that chanting this sound in a predetermined specific way has profound effects on your mind, your voice, the vocal chords, the music that you create, the breathing and the food processing system (chewing, swallowing, filtering, disintegrating and digesting). There actually exists an elaborate scientific explanation. You may be amazed or may be bored to death with the length of the explanation. So, what I do here is present the 'Wikipedia' and

'Google' proofed, and validated facts in point form. I want you to interlink these facts and infer for yourself.

1. A flute, like other wind instruments, produces sound from a vibrating column of air inside the flute. The player makes this column of air vibrate, by blowing air across the top of the flute. The pitch of sound depends on the volume of air that is vibrating. A larger volume vibrates more slowly, producing sound at lower pitch. A smaller volume vibrates more quickly, for brighter pitch. The player changes pitch by opening and closing holes along the flute.

2. You produce sound with your vocal cords and vocal tract having two movements, adduction, i.e., approximation of vocal cords with each other, and abduction, i.e., movement of vocal cords away from each other. The vocal cords (folds) are situated in the voice box (larynx) placed on top of trachea (wind pipe). They have three important functions, to protect airways from choking on material from the throat, to regulate flow of air into lungs and the production of sound for speech.

3. Your wind pipe also works as food pipe. It is a muscular tube running from pharynx to stomach. It transfers the bolus, a moist round partly digested food mass, from mouth to the stomach.

4. The food you consume contains many toxins, adulterants and contaminants. The air you breathe is mostly polluted. The windpipe/food pipe, in conjunction with a few other organs, stops these impurities from entering your lungs and stomach. These impurities get deposited and get leeched on the surface of the food/wind pipe.

5. You clean a dust laden bed sheet, carpet or rug by giving it a violent jerk, by shaking it in air or by vacuum cleaning, thus sucking out the dust.

6. Sound is a vibration. It travels in waveform. It has an amplitude, frequency and a wavelength. This wave returns backwards, reflects and reverberates at a point of discontinuity or at fixed points.

7. When two waves, travelling together or in opposite directions, match in frequency, resonance may occur. Resonance results into waves of much larger amplitude than the original waves.

Now link all these scientific facts and see, if you may produce better sounds and better music, by exercising your vocal chords, in a certain specific way, can you not cleanse and remove leeched impurities by vibrating your wind pipe in a specific way? How will you feel, if you can somehow generate resonance in your wind pipe?

Can you really do it or at least reach a near resonance point? How will your body, mind and internal organs feel, if your food pipe is at or near resonance state? Am I able to make the picture a bit clear? Are you now convinced that by consciously and repeatedly generating some combination of various sounds of a specific nature, you may gain immense benefits for your health? I hope you are at least in the position to grant me the benefits of doubts.

'Ohm' is not a sectarian, religious, eastern centric mantra. It is a universal cosmic sound.

If you are with me so far, let's understand how to create this sound, so beautiful, that our ancestors were tempted to associate it with the God, the creator.

Sit in any comfortable position. 'Sukhasana,' 'Padmasana,' 'Vajrasana' or similar meditation postures are the better ones. You need to take a deep breath, fill your lungs with pure clean air, rich in oxygen. Utilise the additional power of lungs by contracting your hips and pushing the belly skin inwards.

Then, pronounce 'Aum' or 'Ohm' the way as it naturally occurs to you, observing how many different sounds and transitions you are making.

Chances are you would have pronounced it as "OM" the way it is written in a few text books on Yoga. It is the easier way of pronouncing and chanting it. If you counted two sounds of "OOOOH" and "MMMM" with one transition from "O" to "M," you have already got two-thirds of the success. You need to work on the remaining one-third portion only.

Now, chant it the way it is written, "AUM" as long as the air in the lungs allows you to do so. Do not pronounce it as "OM"; you will get only two-thirds of the benefits. Pronounce it as 'AUM!' You need to produce three different sounds, starting with 'AAA…' (sound of Hindi alphabet 'अ') in the beginning, "OOO" (sound of Hindi alphabet 'औ') in the middle and ending with "MMM" (sound of Hindi alphabet 'म'). The time span of each sound should ideally be equal. That means you need to mentally calculate and change the position of your lips. Start with lips relaxed; closed at ends and slightly open in middle; to pronounce 'AAAA.' Then migrate to lips parted fully at centre and forming a circular shape, as close as possible, to pronounce 'OOOO.' And finally reach lips position as closed, tightly at end and loosely at centre to pronounce 'MMMM.'

Tip of the Day

Tip: 'Aum' Recitation for Faster Recollections
'Aum,' is a great sound and a still greater way to acquire instant control over your mind. In your practice sessions, during the learning phase, many a times, difficulties may arise. You may forget your next step or next set of practices. You may even forget 'what you have done so far,' 'what step you were doing' and 'why you were doing it.'
Even when you start your regular Yoga routines, such situation may arise sometimes. Whenever you get into such situation, take a deep breath and start chanting 'AUM.' Simultaneously, mentally try to recollect, 'what step you have just performed' and 'what is the next step.' You should notice that your mental faculties start working better. You are likely to recollect everything much faster.

'Aum' recitation may also be used as a 'filler' for your relaxation phases, in between two set of exercises during the Yoga session. After completing one exercise or asana, while relaxing and regaining normal breathing, recite 'Aum.' This way you may achieve faster and better relaxation as well as recollection of next exercise or asana in the series.

(For Guys). If you have any difficulty in understanding the positioning of your lips for creating three different sounds for chanting 'AUM,' you may better understand it, as lip positions while kissing a girl, your spouse, your girlfriend or whosoever offers her lips to you. You approach for this noble exercise, by keeping your lips closed at ends making a little opening in the middle part of the lips, just enough to prompt her to open-up and offer her lip, upper or lower, depending on your/her choice, for embracing/encasing the lip within your lips. This is the lip formations in first stage.

Once you grab her lip with your lips, you smooch, and caress them by keeping your lips widely parted at centre. This is the second position.

Once the passion gives way to fatigue, she wants to withdraw, but you still want to prolong the moment. So, you apply force to retain her lip, making pressure by closing lips at ends, keeping centre part of lips tightly closed to hang on to holding her lips. This is the third position to pronounce "M."

Now that you know an interesting way to remember your lip positions for creating three different sounds of "AUM," should I not expect you to finish your chant with a 'Muaaah......' sound.

You may also remember these lip positions, by looking at the symbol for Ohm (Ω) the unit for electrical resistance. It is flat in beginning, circular in middle, and flat in end. Of course, there is no 'Muaaah...' in this. After all, it is my creation. Ohm wasn't even aware of this when he created the unit and the symbol.

(For Girls) I hope I haven't hurt your sensibilities by the above statements. Kissing is an expression of love. It is the starting point for continuation of the human race. So why attach any negativity to it.

Now, let us get back to learning!

Sitting in any comfortable posture, take a deep breath. Chant 'ohm' three times, giving a slight pause between two chants and without consciously breathing in between three chants of 'ohm.' Remember, you need to take one deep forceful breath, create nine sounds (three in each chant), six transitions (two in each chant) and two pauses. Try to establish equality in time between 'each chant' and 'each variation of sound.'

No matter what else you do to prepare yourself for your daily Yoga session, you must start your practice by chanting 'Aum' a few times. Better still, chant it the way it is explained. One deep breath! Three chants! Six transitions! Nine different sounds! And two pauses!

While chanting, closely observe the vibrations in your chest from belly to bottom of tongue. They are expected. However, do you expect vibrations on the focal point of your senses? To experience the effect that the chanting has on your brain, place the index finger of right hand softly touching with no exertion of pressure on focal point. You should feel something! If not initially, you will feel it after you complete forty-five days of drill with me. Believe me! It works!

To closely observe the subtle effects that chanting of this innocuous and innocent looking sound makes on your physical, mental and emotional horizons, try the following exercises, in your leisure time.

1. Sitting separately in 'Sukhasana,' 'Ardhpadmasana,' 'Padmasana' and 'Vajrasana,' chant 'Aum' three times after one deep inhalation (three chants, two pauses, nine sounds). Repeat three times in each posture.

2. Repeat this exercise, while focussing attention on the 'Focal point.'

3. Repeat the same exercise focussing attention on the bellybutton.

4. Repeat the same exercise with hands formed in 'Namaskar mudra.'

5. Repeat the same exercise with hands formed in 'Jnana' or 'Chin' mudra.

You may not be able to observe the minute differences in the first instance. Don't lose heart! Believe me, try this exercise, whenever you can spare about thirty minutes. With sustained practice you are likely to observe some funny, pleasant, unexpected, and unbelievable kinds of experiences. Thereafter, you won't disbelieve if some Yoga Guru tells you that he will teach you 'the ways to divine experiences,' 'the methods to unite you with creator' or such similar things. There is nothing great and nothing extraordinary in all such tall claims. There is nothing great in 'divinity.' State of 'pure unadulterated happiness' is divinity.

This chant, you should yourself notice after some practice, generates positive vibes and envelops your complete body, mind, heart and soul in a positive energy capsule. This insulates you from negativities of your surroundings. This makes your meditation work faster and better.

Let me end today's learning by letting you know that once you start seriously practising this chanting, the way it is explained here, you will love my 'Muaaah......' the most. Because, the longer you hold and drag the last sound of 'MMMMM...' the better is the relaxation, immediate fun, sensation and the long-term benefits of the recitation. So always make extra efforts to hold on to the kiss and end it on a happy note. Similarly make extra efforts to keep holding on the last sound of "AUM" and always end it with a 'Muaaah...,' 'Muaaah...,' 'Muaaah...'

Practice for the Day

1. What are you waiting for? There is only one lesson today. Are you waiting for me to prompt you to start practising your 'Ohm' Chanting? Come on! Leave your reservations, if you still have some, and try it! It works!

2. Continue your practice of perfecting the postures of Chapter-One Day-Six to Day-Nine.

Tutorial for the Day

1. Recollect your learning regarding the vibrations, waves and resonance in your wind/food pipe and vocal folds. You might have heard many Yoga teachers making claims to give you the spiritual awakening, divine feelings, to make you one-to-one with the God, to awaken Kundalini, to unlock chakras in your body, and so on. Does it have something to do with achieving resonance during controlled chanting? I am not telling you anything here. Just providing fodder to your thoughts. Explore! Experiment and learn! Do not get guided or misguided by anyone, including me.

Chapter–Two

Day-Thirteen: Mantra Chanting

Learning for the Day

The preachers and practitioners of Yogic art and sciences attach a great significance to chanting mantras. Mantras are generally 'Sanskrit' sentences and phrases, considered sacred in Hindu ways of life. They are difficult to pronounce but generally carry some deeper meanings, wisdom and messages. Your practice session should begin and end with chanting of a few mantras.

I understand your thought process well at this juncture. I know you always doubt my intentions. You may accuse me of going back on my pledges and promises. If others prescribe something and I also do the same, where is the difference? Isn't the belief that chanting some phrases, considered sacred in ancient times will do some good, superstition?

Let me openly confess that I am having equal difficulty in writing these sections, as you are having in assimilating them, with your set of thinking. I also firmly believe that chanting mantras without knowing their meanings, without being aware of the wisdom confined in them and without feeling the message, is sheer stupidity. One may as well sing a song. It will provide better exercise for the vocal cords. It will have more soothing effects on you.

But, if you may somehow feel the hidden message, comprehend the wisdom, and assimilate the meaning of mantra, chanting it should have some positive effect on you. You may also like to recollect your learning from day-eleven. We chanted some chants. They were carrying some meaning and some positive sentences for you. Should you really be that selfish? Should you be thinking of you and you alone? Shouldn't you be thinking of the larger picture?

The nature, the environment, the universe, the humanity and the world peace! Shouldn't you involve these in your thoughts and Yogic practices? Would your chanting for world peace bring peace in the world? No! But maybe it smoothens your guilt feeling. You are at least thinking about it and even praying for it. Others are not even bothered about it. They are just propagating hatred in the name of religion, are indulging in violence and are creating weapons of mass destruction.

Shouldn't the thought, the feeling that you are better than the masses, give you relief, reasons to feel proud and reasons to feel happy? So, why deprive yourself of this wonderful feeling, howsoever miniscule or insignificant, it may be.

May I be permitted to make one suggestion here? Kindly do not allow the strength of your belief systems to be an obstacle in your adoption of Yoga. It is a beautiful science. If you find difficulty in accepting any minor element, a small sub-subject of Yoga, please ignore, leave that sub-topic and move on. But do not leave Yoga as a package. After all, if you notice a small innocuous object floating on your favourite bowl of soup, you will discard the object and not the healthy, tasty, yummy soup.

Involve the larger picture, the greater objectives and some visionary mission statements in your mantras chanting. If you do not find such mantras in the ancient texts or the conventional books, create your own mantras, something having some larger messages and some significant meanings.

For the convenience of the lazy ones, and the ones not blessed with enough creativity to create their own mantras, I am reproducing some mantras for chanting. You must include either your own or a few of these mantras, in the beginning and ending segments of your Yogic routines.

Salutation Mantras

Om Ravaye Namaha, (Salutations to the shining one)

Om Suryaya Namaha, (Salutations to he who induces activity)
Om Bhanave Namaha, (Salutations to he who illumines)

Om Khagaya Namaha, (Salutations to he who moves quickly in the sky)
Om Pushne Namaha, (Salutations to the giver of strength)

Om Hiranya Garbhaya Namaha, (Salutations to the golden, cosmic self)
Om Marichaye Namaha, (Salutations to the Lord of the Dawn)

Om Adityaya Namaha, (Salutations to the son of Aditi, the cosmic Mother)
Om Savitre Namaha, (Salutations to Lord of Creation)

Om Arkaya Namaha, (Salutations to he who is fit to be praised)
Om Bhaskaraya Namaha, (Salutations to he who leads to enlightenment)

Mantra for Peace

Sarve Bhavantu Sukhinaḥ, (May all become happy)
Sarve Santu Nirāmayāḥ (May all be free from all diseases)

Sarve Bhadrāṇi Paśyantu, (May all see the universal truth)
Mākaścit Duḥkha Bhāgbhavet (May no one suffer from any sufferings)

Śāntiḥ! Śāntiḥ!! Śāntiḥ!! (Let there be peace, peace and peace everywhere.
Let there be Universal Peace)

Practice for the Day

1. Continue your practice of perfecting the basic postures of
   Chapter-One. Add 'Aum' recitations and a few mantra chants,
   while practising these postures.

Tutorial for the Day

1. Create your own mantra, song, poem, prose, Tweet, Blog, Facebook-post or any such similar thing, for preaching peace and tranquillity in the world, for eradication of hunger, illiteracy, evils, violence in society, eradication of superstition from the minds of the masses and similar subjects of your likings.

2. 'Gayatri Mantra' is considered most sacred and revered in Hindus' ways of life. Utilise the resources at your command to find out more about this mantra. Set aside your pre-conceived notions and inhibitions and find out why it is considered so sacred by the Hindus.

Chapter–Two

Day-Fourteen: Say Your Prayers

Learning for the Day

In case you are the pious ones, the religious types, and the spiritually enlightened ones and still reading this guide you may skip this section.

Is this the last nail in my coffin? What an irony! A self-confessed atheist asking other atheists, rationalists, logical thinkers, the ones with the scientific temperaments, and the enlightened ones, to pray! Pray to whom and why? Can I really blame anyone else for my plight? After all, it was my decision to preach adoption of Yoga in life to you. I am not going to give up that easily. Here are my efforts to convince you to say some prayers, to eliminate those resistances in your mind.

Saying prayers to the creator, expressing sense of thankfulness and gratitude to your teacher, ability to create the image of the creator in your mind, to enable pointed attention, focus and controls are some of the essential ingredients of Yoga, Meditation and Pranayama. I shall be failing in my duty, if I do not prompt you to derive the best from this beautiful science. Let us tackle this difficult subject, step by step. Let us first resolve the issues of 'Guru/Teacher' and 'God/Creator.'

Adopt a Guru

Why should you adopt a 'Guru'? Pick any book on Yoga, Pranayama, Meditation; they all prescribe you to learn from teachers; from Gurus. You need Gurus to derive the best of benefits of meditation. You need him to say your prayers thanking him, to express your gratitude towards him.

Some may go to the extent of warning you to not attempt any Asana, any posture, any exercises, except under the supervision of a learned Guru.

But, I assured you to be different. I assured you that this is a DIY guide. And look here; I am again prescribing the same medicine for which you discarded other books, other schools and other institutions. So, what is the difference?

Allow me to explain!

You had picked up this book to learn. This means you are interested in learning. You are in quest of knowledge. You purchased this book spending your hard-earned money on it, assuming the knowledge level in this book to be superior to your knowledge level. Knowledge flows from superior to inferior.

Will you go and watch a movie, if you know that the story is inferior to what you can easily write? Visuals are ordinary, what you see daily. The performances are as ordinary as yours in the neighbourhood functions. You go to watch a movie, to experience a superb, complex, and intricate story-line, splendid, grand visuals, beyond your imagination, and extraordinary performances. You go there to satisfy your cravings for creativity. Creativity flows from higher (that of story-writers, director, actors) to lower (you) planes.

Water flows from mountains to lakes, from rivers to seas, from higher heights to lower points. Heat energy transmits from higher temperature to lower temperature. Heat radiates from body of higher temperature to environment at lower temperature. Electrical energy flows from higher to lower potentials. Air flows from higher to lower pressure. So, mass and energy flow automatically from higher planes to lower planes. These are laws of nature.

Knowledge cannot defy the laws of nature. If you need knowledge, 'Gyan,' awareness, enlightenment, you must get it from somewhere up. You need a reference point above you.

That reference point is 'Guru!'

Guru need not be a living human being. In fact, those having gone through their funeral pyre or buried two feet under, are better than those living.

Guru also need not be a human; all you need is an abstract form, a reference point. If your imagination is sharp, creativity strong, so that you can create a form, a reference point, keeping humans a thousand miles away, you are the blessed one. Create him and adopt him.

A few words of cautions here! Note carefully the phrase, 'adopt the Guru.' You need to adopt him, not get adopted by him. You need to use him, and not allow him to use you. You need him for flow of knowledge, not for reverse flow of your wealth. You are the creator, the master.

Many of the modern-day Gurus, the 'Babas,' with mass followings, turned out to be 'Gurughantals' (Hindi word to denote a big-time cheater). Be aware of such Gurus!

Human Gurus invariably are greedy. If not for wealth, they are greedy for promotions. Promotion from human to super-human, super-human to divine, and ultimately to God. You are here in the first place, because you hated the first demon. Now am I asking you to create another? No please! You just need him to serve your purpose. To enable you to derive the best benefits that meditation offers. To soothe certain senses, certain emotions of fulfilment, by saying thanks, and expressing gratitude. If feasible, create him just for those forty-five minutes, just before starting your practice. And allow him to die a natural death, after your practice session is over. Adopt a 'use and throw' Guru.

'Buddha' and 'Ganesha' are ideal forms for adoption. They are familiar. They are nowadays showpieces, visible everywhere. Their form is also good. One is always laughing, and the other seems ever ready to bless you with his trunk. So, instead of any human, better adopt their form.

It shall be best if you can adopt yourself as your Guru. Do you remember those movies, wherein a character, by director's creativity and imagination, gets split into two? The first one, an immaculately dressed person, wearing a white three-piece-suit with white tie and white shoes, acts as morality personified. He is on the right side of everything. The second, a clumsily dressed person, in black tattered clothes, acts as manifestation of all ills. He is on the wrong side of everything. The white and right one tries to persuade and pull the other one to his side. Got the scene!

Now, if you can enact a similar scene and split your personality into two... First, you, the seeker of knowledge, the one in quest, and in hunger of peace and tranquillity. Second, the other you, the learned, enlightened one, ever ready to part with knowledge for others' benefit. You, 'the first one' can adopt you 'the second one' as your ('the first one's) Guru. This may sound difficult, but best results with no risks are guaranteed.

I hope I have been able to sell my theory of adoption.

Yogic practices require you to make and to create an image of Guru in your mind, to honestly, diligently and obediently follow his instructions, to focus your senses on the Guru's image, to say thanks to him in prayers, to express gratitude, to leave yourself at his command, to have trust and faith on him.

Please do not create resistance in the above for your own benefit. Adopt a 'Guru!'

Assume a Creator

I am encouraged in writing this book, as despite being a staunch atheist, I adopted Yoga after lots of hits and trials, failures and re-attempts, resistances and acceptances, and experimentations and observations. You picked up this book to learn Yoga, without compromising your beliefs, without conceding defeat in debate on existence of God and without believing that 'Brahma,' 'Vishnu,' 'Mahesh,' 'Kailasha,' 'Paigamber,''Jesus,' 'Allah,' 'Beths' or 'Moses' has any role in creation. And look here; both of us are discussing about the creator, the God.

Have faith in me! I have no intention of changing your beliefs. At the end of this book, I intend to leave you with enhanced knowledge on Yoga only. You may by default strengthen some of your knowledge on science. We need this concept, this abstract form of creator for exactly the same purpose as Gurus, but on a much higher plane. In fact, on topmost planes, we want him at infinity.

In an earlier part of this book, I attempted convincing you to assume nature to be the creator. If you are comfortable with this hypothesis, it is absolutely fine. It serves the intended purpose and nothing more is required.

The problem that may arise is, assigning a form to nature. A form needed for a reference point at infinity, in eternity, the supreme form. We generally envision nature as a canvass of mountains, castles, rivers, deserts, land, seas, fountains, flowers, animals, birds, etc. etc. Unless you are an accomplished painter, it is difficult to paint this canvass in your imagination, establish it in your mind, and keep your mind unwaveringly focussed on it.

For God's sake (pun intended) do not assume the creator in any form even remotely similar to humans. We need an abstract concept and not a substitute.

If you are comfortable, you may substitute the concept with someone you believe to be more important than you, in your life. He/she may be a girlfriend, a wife or a parent. So, when asked to focus, to tie your brain, your mind with leash to God, you may instead, tie it to her/him.

You may also choose your idol, if you have one, your favourable movie star or starlet, though I personally discourage this. Your idol, that favourite star of yours is in no way superior to you. He may turn out to be much lower in intelligence, in knowledge, and may be even in looks and performance skills. You must believe in yourself, have confidence in yourself. You are better than others. You are the best.

Your favourite star, your idol, after enjoying many, many years of your adulation and your admiration, may later turn out to be a crook, a rapist, a murderer, a fraudster and in most cases a tax-evader. Such situations cause avoidable emotional disturbance and stresses. They are best avoided by treating all human beings as what they actually are, as either equal or inferior to you.

My sincere advice is for not allowing, not allocating any space above you to anyone else, except the 'adopted Guru' and the 'assumed creator.' There are just three of you in this universe, Guru on a pedestal slightly above you, enveloping you, forming an impregnable shield of protection all around you, showering his acquired wisdom, his knowledge on you, and the assumed creator, blessing you, bestowing the peace, tranquillity and the happiness on you.

Imagine the scene! Feel the protection! Enjoy the release! Enjoy the contentment! Enjoy the happiness! Enjoy the learning! Enjoy the knowledge! Enjoy the enlightenment! Enjoy…enjoy and enjoy!

Relax…! Relax…!! and… Relax!!!

Saying Your Prayers

I have put you through all these pains, these trials and turbulences, tensions, compressions and stresses on all your resistance levels, for a single purpose. So that you may say, sing, recite, and chant your prayers with comfort and convictions during meditation.

Why Should You Pray?

You should pray, because prayers have immense powers.

- The powers of positive-auto-suggestions.
- The powers of a support system, to fall back upon, when in need, stress, or distress.

- The powers of assumption of a protective shield around you.

- The powers of controlling your mind to enable it to rest, refrain from anfractuous wanderings, refresh and rejuvenate. Conserve precious blood, water, oxygen and energy that are wasted in such fruitless activities. It is the biggest consumer of all your internal resources. Conservation here is very important.

- The prayers have powers to tell your heart, that all is well.

So, if prayers are so powerful why shouldn't we leave atheism? Pray to God and be happy. And hey! Why is it that the priest 'Pujariji' is not the happiest, healthiest man on earth?

We are atheist by choice and by our convictions, that there is no God. No one, in human form needs to be credited and kept pleased by prayers, for being associated with creation. We will believe, what science tells us to be true, and nothing else. Prayers, for personal wealth, for that promotion that you desire and do not deserve, are simply futile. Prayers for universal peace are not. Prayers for eradication of superstition are not.

Prayers may not bring peace in universe, but will give you a little solace, a satisfaction, that you did your bit for it. You even prayed. You know, mere prayers can achieve nothing, leave alone the universal peace. You must do a lot more for it. You also must do a lot more to achieve personal health, peace, satisfaction, contentment and happiness.

So why don't we begin by saying some prayers.

Hey creator! Accept my salutation and gratitude. I bow, before you. Please give me your blessings.	हे सृष्टि-रचयिता! आभार! प्रणाम! चरण वंदना। कृपया आशीर्वाद दें।
Hey teacher! I salute you. Kindly bless me with knowledge.	

<table>
<tr>
<td>

I am going to start learning Yoga. I am going to start my Yoga practice. Kindly bless me. Kindly grant me the wisdom.

Kindly allow all my senses to focus on my learning. Kindly allow all my attention on the focal point of all my senses. Let there be no distractions.

So, help me the Creator. So, help me the Guru.

</td>
<td>

हे गुरूवर प्रणाम । कृपया शुभाशीष दें। मैं योगाभ्यास के लिए बैठ रहा हूं। कृपया कृपादृष्टि बनाए रखें।
मेरा ध्यान कहीं भी इधर-उधर ना भटके।
मेरा समस्त ध्यान मेरे इन्द्रियों के केन्द्र-बिन्दु पर केन्द्रित रहे।

</td>
</tr>
</table>

Let all my attention be focussed on the focal point of all my senses.
Let all my attention be focussed on the focal point of all my senses.
Let all my attention be focussed on the focal point of all my senses.
Let all my attention be focussed on the focal point of all my senses.
Let all my attention be focussed on the focal point of all my senses.

Look carefully at the paragraph above. There is a purpose in writing the above phrase, the way it is written. While chanting, start saying the phrase loudly, simultaneously asking your brain to focus on the focal point, eyes to point towards the central point of eyebrows, ears and nose to be attentive towards the focal point. Keep on reducing the sound levels, the way font size is being reduced in repeated chanting. This way, it is easier to attain focus.

You may create your own prayers, your own recitation, involving senses of thankfulness and gratitude to teachers, love, affection and surrender to creator with positive vibes, positive energies, positive thoughts and suggestions. And yes, remember no begging and no bargaining before the creator! Remember, you only created him.

The gates to meditation have just been opened, with a 'welcome' mat and a red carpet waiting for your arrival.

Welcome to the blissful world of meditation, the most powerful arm of Yoga.

Day-Fifteen: Basics of Meditation Practices

Learning for the Day

Hey! Congratulations! You have learnt the postures, the 'Aum' and 'Mantra' chanting and saying your prayers. And most important! You have surpassed the most important hurdles of not having a Guru and a Lord. You deserve a huge round of applause, for tolerating me for more than fourteen days now. I know, it was tough on you. It was equally difficult for me too. But rest assured! I shall be far better from the next section onwards. Your learning shall be much more enjoyable.

Now that you have learnt the essential elements of meditation, you are ready to start practising meditation, the most important limb of Yoga. So, I will now teach you the techniques of meditation.

Meditation is nothing! Yes! Meditation is nothing! Doing nothing is meditating.

So, what do I teach when there is nothing to teach? These, gentlemen are the harsh realities of meditation, the art.

No matter whosoever makes whatsoever claims, no one can teach you meditation. Only you can teach meditation to yourself.

Sitting in comfortable posture, for long hours, breathing normally, saying some prayers, chanting some mantras and thus focussing all your senses, attention and energies at one point, is simply put, meditation. All I can do to guide you further, is to summarise the essential learning from Chapter-Two. Here is the summary:

Posture

You may sit in any comfortable position. 'Padmasana,' though a bit difficult, is considered the best position. You may initially sit in 'Sukhasana' or 'Ardhpadmasana' and try 'Padmasana' and other advanced Asanas (there are many more, not covered in this guide) after some days of practice. You may also meditate sitting on a chair, in 'Vajrasana,' 'Tadasana,' or any other posture, as long as you are bodily comfortable and may allow your brain to focus and concentrate and keep the posture steady.

The basic purpose of the Meditation Asanas is to facilitate sitting for longer durations of time, keeping the body steady and comfortable. Only when the body remains still and steady for long times, the effects of meditation will be experienced. Deep meditation requires the spinal column to be straight. Very few sitting postures (Asanas) can satisfy this condition.

Further, in high stages of meditation, the practitioner may lose control over the muscles of the body. The meditation asana, therefore, needs to hold the body in a steady position without conscious effort.

The logical query that may arise here is 'Why not lie in Shavasana, then, for meditation, since it satisfies all the requirements?' This is because, in Shavasana the practitioner may drift into sleep. It is essential to remain awake and alert while going through the various stages which lead one to achieve success and derive benefits from meditation.

"You must be able to sit in one of the Meditation Asanas for a full three hours at a stretch without the body shaking. Then only will you gain true 'asana siddhi' mastery over the asana and be able to practise the higher stages of Pranayama and dhyana. Without securing a steady asana you cannot progress well in meditation. The more steady you are in your asana, the more you will be able to concentrate with a one-pointed mind. If you can be steady in a posture even for one hour, you will be able to acquire a one-pointed

*mind and feel the 'atmic anandam,' infinite peace and soulful bliss
inside you."*

*– Swami Sivananda of Rishikesh,
Uttrakhand, India*

Before Starting

Some selected 'Sukshma-Vyayama' practices from the 'Pawanamuktasana'
series are useful for loosening of stiff joints and preparing the body for
the Meditation Asanas. Half butterfly (Ardh-titali-asana), hip rotations
(Shroni chakra), full butterfly (Poorna-titali-asana), abdominal stretch
poses, etc., may be performed prior to starting. (Refer Chapter-Four) Start
with three to four cycles of 'Aum' recitations, a few mantra chanting and
saying a prayer.

Mind and Brain

Focussed on one point, one issue and one agenda. If possible create/
paint an image of the creator and/or a Guru, establish this image in your
brain (at focal point of all senses) and let your brain focus on this image.
The left part of brain, the creative one, should be in the most creative
state. The right brain at its logical best. Concentration and focus is
the key.

You may try and programme the mind to make suggestions like,
"I am as steady as a rock" or "I am becoming motionless like a statue." This
way the asana will quickly become steady and, after some time, it will feel
comfortable for extended periods of time

Eyes

Best to be shut, closed, viewing the image of the Lord/Guru in your mind.
If closing eyes not practical, mark a reference point on the front wall and
focus eyes on this point alone.

Hands

Best in Namaskar Mudra, or placed on respective knees, in 'Jnana' or 'Chin' Mudra. Arms loose or slightly stretched.

Breathing

Normal, through nostrils, unlaboured, unforced.

All Limbs

Comfortable, steady and at ease.

Do's

Sit comfortably. Concentrate. Focus. Nothing else. If mind wavers, take a deep breath, chant 'AUM' and bring it back to focus. Allow everything else to wait. This is your time. Enjoy it. Deadlines can wait! Death-lines don't. The time to postpone the deadlines for postponing the death-line is now! Targets are for you! You are not for the targets! Relax! Relax!! And Relax!!!

Only if severe discomfort or pain in the legs is felt after sitting for some time, slowly unlock the legs and massage them. When the blood circulation returns to normal and pain subsides, resume the asana. Beware that the knee is a delicate and much abused joint of the body. So, be careful not to overstrain it, especially while moving into or out of the postures.

To smoothen long sitting it is better to place a small cushion under the buttocks.

Don'ts

Feel stretched. Feel stressed. Desire. Aspire. Worry. Fear. Remember any task, target or timelines. Listen to any unpleasant, distracting sounds. Look at watch for time.

Practice for the Day

1. Sitting in any comfortable posture, meditate for fifteen minutes. Do not put any undue stress or strain on any part of your body, mind and heart system. Do nothing during these fifteen minutes. At the end of the time consider what all thoughts came to your mind. If possible, make a list. Ponder how you can overcome, overpower and overrule your mind, so that no unwanted thinking occurs.

2. Make a holistic assessment of your needs and expectations from Yoga, for developing your routines for daily practices. Assess how much time you need to assign for meditation. This time should be commensurate with your stress levels, emotional turbulences, negativities and depression in life.

Chapter-Three

Pranayama

Day-Sixteen: Breathing for Fun

Learning for the Day

Breathing is life. To breathe is to live. Breathing gone, life over! You are breathing, so you are living. You want to live, so you must breathe. You want to live better, so you must breathe better. Simple!

You haven't been blessed with life to carry the weight of this world on your shoulders. You are not existing in this universe to work and slog like a donkey. You have not been dispatched to this beautiful mother earth to bear all the stresses. To work for living is a requisite, not the purpose of life. Stress is an unnecessary, avoidable evil, stuck with a strong adhesive with life.

Work pressures and stresses are like those useless birthday and anniversary gifts you receive from friends and relatives. Even in your wildest imagination and with the best of creativity, you find no use for them. You must live with them, make space and keep them in your house, till you find an appropriate occasion to pass them on to some other useless relative. Work and stress is for passing on to others. Life is to enjoy, have fun!

Breathing is life. Life is for fun. So why shouldn't we start our learning of 'Pranayama' with some fun. Let's have some fun with our breathing.

Your body needs oxygen. Plenty of it! You are fortunate that despite our (the human being's) best efforts to destroy all oxygen, there is still some left in the air. It is just twenty to twenty-one per cent. It is just enough for you and me to breathe and to survive. Unless we, you and I, do something, there will be none left for others. May be none left, even for those little bundles of joy, we call as our children. So, let us make the optimum use of this precious resource. Breathe proper! Let your body give the best mileage with this costly fuel.

To inhale, retain and exhale air, is breathing. There are air filters in your body, ensuring only clean air enters your body. In fact, there are pre-filters, filters, micro-filters and nano-filters. There are other organs which take oxygen and digest your food, convert solids and liquids into energy. There are other organs to produce blood, and to purify blood, all requiring oxygen.

When you deprive your body of air, or supply dirty, impure, unclean air, all these organs curse you. They slow down their functioning. There is another set of supply-chain-manager organs, which send distress signals, of low supply of oxygen and impending doom, all around. Result— crisis in body, fire-fighting, top management howling at full throttle, middle management running all around, doing nothing, but showing hyper-activity to bosses. The working class gets all stressed, fatigued, and fearful of firing, job-loss, pay-cuts, no increments, etc. Familiar with the scene! Well similar crisis occurs in your body, day in and day out, thousands of times in a day. Only gravity of crisis varies.

If you are not familiar with organisational functioning and can't make head or tail of the above paragraphs, imagine shortages of critical food items, say grains, salt or sugar, with all markets closed due to indefinite curfew in your city.

On the other hand, whenever abundant, clean, pure, oxygen-rich air is made available, all these oxygen dependent organs rejoice. They party, as if there is no tomorrow. The logistics team, the store keepers, all give positive vibes; send 'all-available' signals to all and sundry. Top management starts thinking of new orders. Middle management is content and happy, there is less pressure to conserve, produce more with lesser raw materials.

The working class feels happy. Everyone dreams of bonus, pay raise, increment, paid holidays. Trust me! Your body is a more complex organisation than you may imagine. And oxygen is the most important raw material it processes.

You generally inhale through your nose. You also generally, without knowing about it, exhale through your nose. Your nose contains two nostrils, two openings for inhalations and exhalations. Both, as you can see, are equal in size. Both should play equal role, share the equal work, equal burden, and equal pressure in both exhalations and inhalations. (Do they? We will learn later!)

You can also take in air through your mouth. Inhale through mouth. You can also exhale through your mouth. If you are a gym enthusiast, a runner, sportsman, athlete, or have recently made a run to catch a bus, train or second glimpse of that beautiful girl or handsome guy, who hurriedly crossed you in that busy market, you should know that your breathing becomes faster, laboured and forceful in such situations.

You also unknowingly tend to breathe through your mouth. Inferences drawn: you can suck in more oxygen through your mouth than your nose. Your body, working under the command and control of your mind, automatically makes a switchover and starts breathing through mouth, your nose taking rest.

You have two respiratory systems. First, through nose, which is the default system; whether you ask it or not, it will do its work. And second, through the mouth, the emergency system, the reserve, gets automatically activated, when the default organ is not able to handle the work.

You have three openings, three inlets and three outlets in your body for inhalation and exhalations. Right! Oh no! There is one more, only outlet for...but that is not exhalations! Come on man! You are dirty.

Exercises for the Day

Fun Breathing Exercise Number 1: Inhale and Exhale through Nose

Steps:

- Remember and follow the prerequisites.

- Sit in any relaxation or meditation posture, brain focussed on focal point, eyes closed. Ears should be receptive to only sounds of silence, soft music, chirping of birds, humming of bees, breeze, flowing water, and closed for all other sounds. Body be at rest and loose.

- Hands hung loosely hinged on shoulders! Both arms resting on legs! Legs folded in 'Sukhasana,' 'Ardhpadmasana' or 'Padmasana!' Bottom of palm touching knees! Palm loose, fingers in Jnana Mudra!

- Hold yourself in this posture and relax!

- Perform meditation for at least five minutes. Chant 'Aum,' some mantras and say some prayers.

- Breathe in through your nose and breathe out through nose slowly. Count. Do not exert any pressure, any tension, any stretching on any organ! Simply breathe in through nose and breathe out through nose, counting each exhalation and each inhalation. Count to forty. Twenty inhalation and twenty exhalations.

- Now, close one of the nostrils by pressure of finger and thumb and breathe through another open nostril. Count to twenty. Repeat by closing the second nostril. Count to twenty. Are both nostrils behaving in identical manner and sharing equal burden?

- Notice that the breath is cool when it enters the nostrils and warm when it flows out.

- Relax! Relax! and Relax!

- Let's call this exercise for the sake of remembrance as "**Nose-in-Nose-out.**" For easy recall give it a nickname **Ni-No** (Nose in, Nose out).

Fun Breathing Exercise Number 2: Inhale and Exhale through Mouth

Steps:

- Repeat the above exercise giving complete rest to your nose and inhaling and exhaling through mouth. Count forty (20–20).

- Try the following variations for both inhalations and exhalations.

  a. Open your mouth only slightly. Lips should open slightly in the middle, the gaps between lips tapering down from middle to sideways. Inhale, exhale, count, do not make any sound.

  b. Now form a circle with your lips. Use a circular opening of your mouth for breathing, making a whistling sound. If you are an expert whistler or know whistling, make as loud a sound of whistle in both inhalation and exhalation as you can. Keep on counting. Count forty. Enjoying! Feeling good!! Having fun!

- Relax! Relax! and Relax!

- Let us call this as **Mouth-in-Mouth-Out (Mi-Mo).**

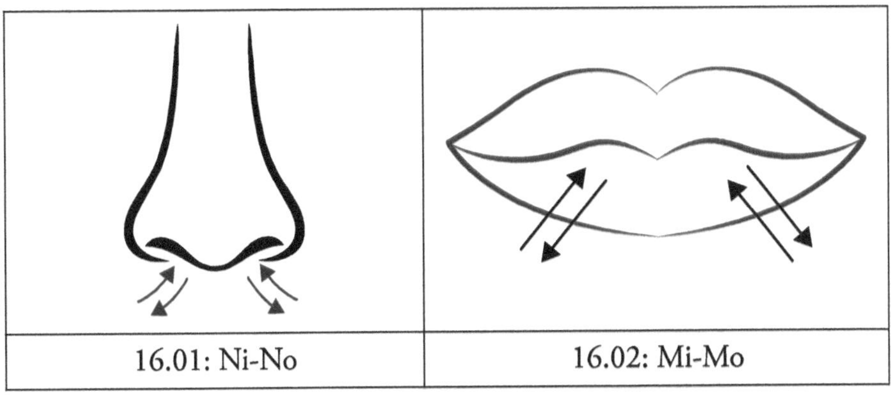

16.01: Ni-No	16.02: Mi-Mo

Fun Breathing Exercise Number 3: Cross Breathings, Inhale through Nose and Exhale Through Mouth

Steps:

- Repeat the same exercise crossing your breathings, inhaling through nose and exhaling through mouth. Count forty (20–20).

- During exhalation perform whistling, if you like.

- Let us call this as **Nose-in-Mouth-Out (Ni-Mo).**

Fun Breathing Exercise Number 4: Cross Breathings, Inhale through Mouth and Exhale Through Nose

Steps:

- Repeat the same exercise crossing your breathings, and reversing the actions, i.e., inhaling through mouth and exhaling through nose. Count forty (20–20).

- During inhalation perform whistling, if you like.

- Let us call this as **Mouth-In-Nose-Out (Mi-No).**

These four exercises, serve the purpose of warming up, in preparing you for performing 'Pranayama' exercises. Now let us try some more fun breathing exercises involving holding of breath, i.e., prolonging the retention period of breath inside the belly.

Fun Breathing Exercise Number 5: Holding the Breath

Steps:

- Breathe in through your nose, mentally calculating the time taken in inhalation. Now, when your lungs and belly are filled with air, hold your breath, for roughly the same time that you took in inhalation, or for as long as you find it comfortable. Thereafter, release the breath and breathe out through nose slowly and normally. Count.

- Do not exert any pressure, any tension, any stretching on any organ! Simply breathe in through nose, hold and breathe out through nose. Counting each exhalation and each inhalation, count to forty, twenty inhalations and twenty exhalations.

- Let us call this as **Nose-In-Hold-Nose-Out routine (Ni-Ho-No).**

- You may similarly perform the **Mouth-in-Hold-Mouth-Out (Mi-Ho-Mo), Nose-In-Hold-Mouth-Out (Ni-Ho-Mo)** and **Mouth-in-Hold-Nose-Out (Mi-Ho-No)** routines.

That was good! Wasn't it? Did you try whistling, while inhaling or exhaling through mouth? Aren't the nicknames that we are assigning to each routine, interesting? Are you enjoying doing the stuff? Having fun! Now let's add some more spice to the fun. Let us try some forceful breathing-ins.

Fun Breathing Exercise Number 6: Forced Breathings

Steps:

You may force your inhalations, through nose by three ways:

- Utilising power of your lungs, after normal intake of air in, apply your lung power to suck some more air in.

- After having filled your lungs with as much air as they can hold, pause and contract your hips, utilising the powers of hip muscles, push in the two halves of buttocks, towards the centre, closer to each other, closing the opening as far as possible. By this deliberate gesture, you may squeeze in some more air.

- Hold on, it is not over yet. There are still spaces inside your belly that you may fill in with air. You can do this by forcefully tucking in your belly. Apply the force of your tummy muscles and pull the front skin backwards, towards the back. This way a small cavity gets formed around your navel area. This action helps in pumping in some more air.

- Now understand that you must do this forceful inhalation in a smooth and jerk-free manner. Transition from one stage to another should be smooth. Do not give unnecessary pauses in between. Do not overdo things. Apply only as much force as comfortable. Understand the sequence.

  1. Breathe in normally.

  2. Apply lungs power, sucking in some more air.

  3. Apply hips muscle power, contract hips and pump in some more air.

  4. Now activate and unlock the powers of stomach muscles and squeeze in belly, taking some more air in the last attempt.

Do I need to tell you, that if I denote forceful inhalation with 'Fo,' you may try the following routines?

- **Nose-in-Forced-Nose-out (Ni-Fo-No) routine.**

- **Nose-in-Forced-Mouth-Out (Ni-Fo-Mo) routine.**

- **Nose-In-Forced-Hold-Nose-Out (Ni-Fo-Ho-No) routine.**

- **Nose-In-Forced-Hold-Mouth-Out (Ni-Fo-Ho-Mo) routine.**

Fun Breathing Exercise Number 7: Exhalations Only

Just for fun and enhancing your awareness of your own breaths try out the followings also:

- Exhale only slowly, without bothering about inhalations. Inhalation will occur naturally. Do not make any attempt at retention also. Decide a pace of say about one exhalation per second and exhale slowly.

- Increase the intensity of exhalation reducing speed correspondingly. Again, do not make any conscious efforts towards inhalations or retention. Allow these to occur naturally.

- Place your palm in front of mouth at one to two inches away from mouth, to judge the temperature of air being expelled during exhalations. Exhale slowly through mouth, expelling only the air trapped in portions of body above neck. Increase the intensity of exhalations, consciously making efforts, to expel the air from the portion of body between head and stomach. Now again increase force in exhalations, to consciously expel the air in belly region. Observe the difference in temperatures in the three different variants of exhalations.

Try these one by one, making just one attempt at one routine, else you will get tired. Enjoyed them? These are great exercises for warming up your system. Please note that in these exercises your mind, focus and attention, etc., were not involved. Your brain was free to indulge in activities of his own liking.

These exercises were at physical levels only. After some more learning, when you start real Pranayama exercises, the action and inactions of mind, attention and focus will play a much greater role. To appreciate the difference better, you may later perform both the fun breathing exercises and corresponding Pranayama exercise during some leisurely days. It may prove to be an eye opener for you.

These exercises have been carefully crafted to enhance your awareness on breathing and to smoothly lead you towards Pranayama. Otherwise these are just fun exercises and may at best be used to warm up and prime the body and mind for the real 'Pranayama' exercises. Initially in your learning phase you must include a few of these in your package of daily practices.

Once you become expert, there is not much need to perform them on daily basis. However, they are great fun routines. You may make a package, a sequence of exercises, make a chart of the acronyms, and paste it on a wall in front of you. This way you may easily complete the package of exercises. Complete one routine; see what comes next, by merely glancing at the chart and seeing a few alphabets, i.e., Ni-Mo, Mi-No, you will come to know what is next. **Wasn't it fun so far!**

Chapter–Three

Day-Seventeen: Basics of Pranayama

Learning for the Day

The Meanings

An immature attempt to understand the literal meaning of the 'Hindi' word 'Pranayama' may erroneously result in quite dangerous interpretations. It is a combination of two words 'Prana' and 'Yama.' 'Prana' literally translates into "life." 'Pranavayu' means life breath. 'Yama' in Hindu philosophy is the 'Lord of Death.' A fellow carrying an image of a human with two large pointed horns on his head, wearing black robes and riding on his favourite mode of transport, the male buffalo. He is supposed to take the life breath and the soul away to another world in 'Hell' or 'Heaven' once the life's last innings is over. Dangerous subject! Isn't it? So, why should you study and practise this dangerous thing, connected with death?

What if I give you another positive interpretation? It is the Art and Science of ensuring 'Prana' does not reach 'Yama' so fast. Interested! Now, let us understand the actual meaning. 'Pranayama' literally means 'regulation of breath.' The 'breath' here is not the physical breathing alone. It has a much larger and wider meaning, which we will slowly understand. In 'Pranayama'; fresh air is inhaled, and foul air is exhaled, in a regulated manner. The breath literally acts as a carrier of vital force or 'Prana.'

'Pranayama' also literally means **'to expand Prana'** (Vital force) or to expand the life span. Pranayama is a process in which respiration is interrupted and 'Prana,' that is, 'the vital force' is controlled and regulated. The purpose of 'Pranayama' is to inspire, motivate, regulate and balance the vital force ('Prana'), (the sources of various energies, physical and metaphysical) prevailing in the body. It is the soul of Yoga. In a nutshell, some proper balances of inhalations, exhalations and retention are the key points of 'Pranayama.'

The Advantages

- Keeps the body oxygenated, fit and healthy.

- Reduces excessive fat.

- One can live a longer life through 'Pranayama.'

- Improves the power of memory and eliminates mental disorders.

- Tones up the stomach, the liver, the bladder, the small and the large intestines and the digestive system, purifies tubular channels and removes sluggishness from the body, and kindles gastric fire; the body becomes healthy and the inner voice begins to be heard.

- Constant practice strengthens the nervous system. The mind becomes calm and capable of concentration.

- Negative thinking comes to an end. The person practising Pranayama is always full of positive thoughts.

The Prerequisites

The prerequisites for practising the Pranayama are the same as before. Do recollect your learnings of Chapters One and Two, if required. The postures suitable are 'Sukhasana,' 'Ardhpadmasana,' 'Padmasana,' 'Siddhasana,' or 'Vajrasana.' In case you have not yet perfected your postures, in the beginning, you may sit erect on a chair. Keep the spine fully vertical and stretched.

Casual smokers may experience frequent and may be forceful coughing in the initial phases. Do not worry! This is normal and part of the cleansing and detoxification of lungs and respiratory system. If you are suffering from mild cold, cough or chest congestion, start practising slower versions. Do keep a hand towel or a box of tissues handy, to wipe out the nasal discharges. Even otherwise, it should make sense to keep a towel or tissues handy.

Important Steps in Pranayama and Terminology

You need to understand and grasp certain important steps of 'Pranayama' and the terms used, which are as follows. I am constrained in using some difficult Sanskrit words here, so that you are not found wanting in your interactions with a trained practitioner.

- 'Puraka' means 'Inhaling.'

- 'Kumbhaka' is the 'retention of the breath.'

- 'Rechaka' means 'Exhaling.'

- 'Puraka' (means to inhale), 'Kumbhaka' (means to retain the breath) and 'Rechaka' (means to exhale) completes one cycle of breathing, i.e., one breath.

- 'Bandhas' are the carefully crafted, forceful exercises either to enable prolongation of inhaling (forceful effort to inhale more than normal air) or forceful retention of air after inhalation. These are like applying locks on the air passages.

- There are three 'Bandhas' (locks), i.e., 'Jalandhar Bandha,' 'Uddiyana Bandha,' and 'Moola Bandha.'

- 'Bahya' (External) 'Kumbhaka' means 'retention of breath after exhalation.'

- 'Antarika' (Internal) 'Kumbhaka' means retention of breath following inhalation.

Bandhas

These 'Bandhas' are extremely beneficial in Pranayama. 'Bandhas' means 'to block' or 'to stop.' We put a lock (block) to that outgoing energy (Aura) of the body and organs, which we wish to utilise for our inner body through 'Pranayama.' There are three Bandhas (blocks). Note: The subject of Bandha may look intimidating and complex initially. You are advised to link it to the theoretical parts of 'Hasta-Mudra' and practical aspects of fun breathing exercises for better understanding.

1. Jalandhar Bandha

Techniques:

- Sitting erect in 'Vajrasana,' 'Padmasana' or 'Siddhasana,' take a long breath out and hold.

- Put both hands on respective knees, 'in jnana mudra.' First stretch your neck slightly upwards and immediately thereafter lower your chin towards the hollow in the throat ('kanthakula'). This posture is known as 'Jalandhar Bandha.' This Bandha blocks the network of the throat.

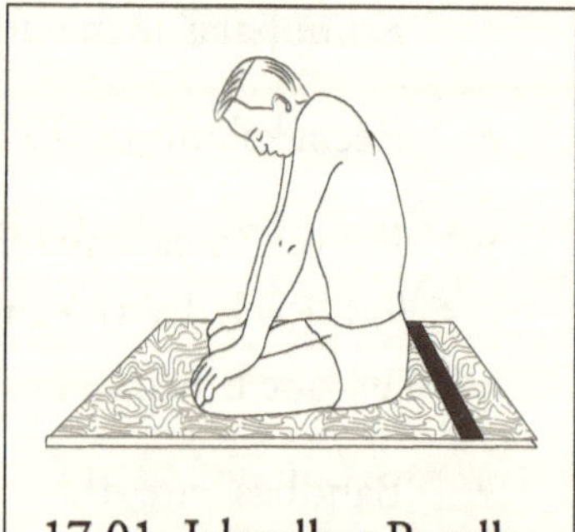

17.01: Jalandhar Bandha

- The parts around the throat including the thyroid gland are pressed in this Bandha; the back portion of the neck is stretched. An upward pull is exercised on the spine.

- This Bandha is not to be applied during 'Puraka' (Inhalation) or 'Rechaka' (Exhalation).

- This Bandha should always accompany 'Kumbhaka,' either 'Bahya' (External) or 'Antrika' (Internal).

Benefits:

- This Bandha leads to sweet, soft and musical throat.

- It is a healer of almost all the throat problems and very much beneficial for the problems associated with Thyroid and Tonsils.

2. Uddiyan Bandha

Techniques:

- In this Bandha, the thoracic diaphragm (around the navel region) is moved to an extreme upward position.

- The wall of the abdomen is pulled towards the back giving a concave appearance like the bottom surface of a pond. That is usually done after an exhalation so that the depression in the wall of the abdomen looks quite pronounced.

- When it is done while holding the breath in, during 'Pranayama' the concavity is not so well marked

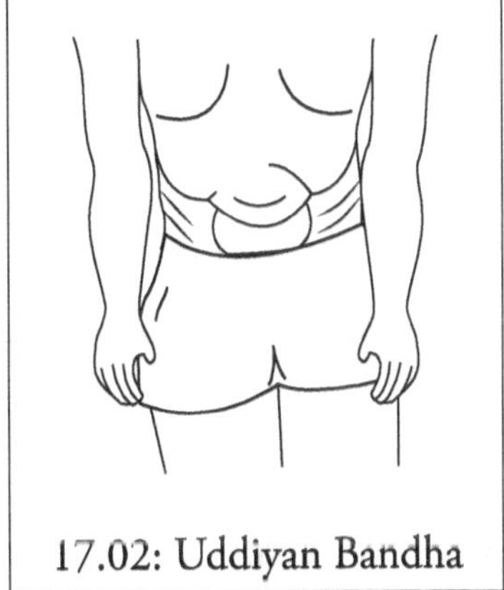

17.02: Uddiyan Bandha

because the diaphragm does not rise high in the thoracic cavity since the lungs are already filled with air.

Benefits:

- This Bandha provides a very good exercise to the abdominal viscera by causing pressure and stretch on them.

- This helps to remove congestion and promotes blood circulation. While doing it in 'Pranayama' after a 'puraka' (inhaling), a stretch and pressure is developed in both the thoracic and abdominal cavities.

3. Moola Bandha

'Moola' means the root. 'Moolabandha' is the contraction of the anal sphincters and the pelvic floor. While in 'Uddiyanabandha' one sucks the belly in, the lower abdomen is also slightly contracted. This contraction is completed by contracting the anal sphincters. Thus 'Uddiyanbandha' and 'Moolabandha' usually go together.

Techniques:

- Either by sitting in 'Vajrasana,' 'Siddhasana' or 'Padmasana,' take a long breath out and hold.

- Consciously pull both the anus and the penis upward, the lower part of the navel will automatically be stretched upward. Two halves of buttocks will also automatically come closer to each other.

Benefits:

- This Bandha heals constipation, piles, and stimulates the system.

- It provokes the semen to travel upward and is most important for the maintenance of celibacy, if one is interested.

4. Maha Bandha

By sitting in any meditation, concentrative asana like 'Vajrasana,' 'Padmasana,' 'Siddhasana' or 'Sukhasana,' applying all the three Bandhas at the same time is known as 'Mahabandha.'

In this posture, hips are contracted, belly skin pressed inwards, and respiratory passage is closed by pulling chin downwards and allowing chin to touch the skin of your chest, according to capacity.

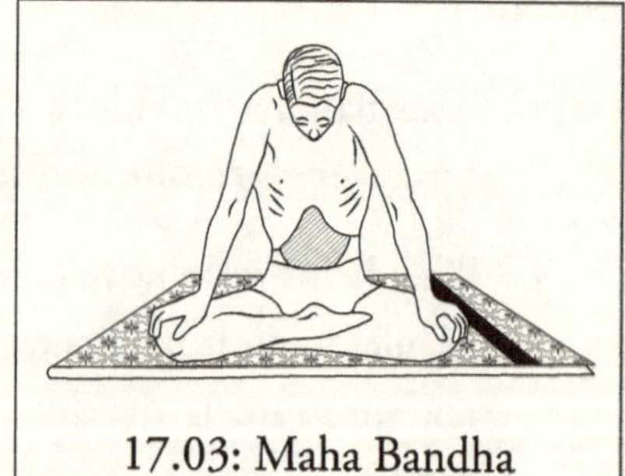

17.03: Maha Bandha

This Bandha is to be performed in 'Kumbhak' (retention of breath) state. It can be performed with 'Bahya' (External) 'Kumbhaka' (retention of breath after exhalation) or with 'Antarika' (Internal) 'Kumbhaka' (retention of breath following inhalation).

Practice for the Day

1. Continue some fun breathing exercises. Practise all three Bandhas.

2. Recollect your learning of hands formations (Hasta-Mudras'). Link it to current subject of 'Bandhas.' Recollect the energy block principles. You shall be practising some Bandhas and Mudras very soon.

Day-Eighteen: Easy, Effective, Everyday Pranayama: Part – I

Learning and Practice for the Day

This section includes some easy and most effective 'Pranayama' techniques. The 'Pranayama' in this section are of 'must perform' and 'must include' kinds. Irrespective of the duration of your daily routine Yoga practice, minimum two or all Pranayama of this section, each for duration of two to five minutes must be included in daily routines for better results.

Bhastrika Pranayama

Precautions:

- Patients of Asthma should not practice it.

- Persons suffering from high blood pressure and heart problems should only do slow 'Bhastrika' and preferably under the care of a specialist.

- Do take special care of your dentures during forced exhalation. They should not experience an unnecessary jerk.

- Persons with common cold and sinus infection and clogged nostrils may first clear their nasal passage with 'Jalaneti.' (A Yogic practice of cleaning the nasal passage with water by squeezing in water in one nostril and oozing it out from another nostril).

- While practising 'Pranayama' process the eyes should be closed and every breath, either inhaling or exhaling should be mingled with the thought of 'OHM,' or 'AUM' or some other similar symbol.

Technique:

- Sit in any meditative posture at ease. Filling the lungs with breath through nostrils and throwing it out through nostrils only, with full force is called 'Bhastrika' Pranayama.

- The abdominal cavity moves like a balloon in 'Bhastrika.' See 18.01: (State during inhalation) and 18.02: (State during exhalation).

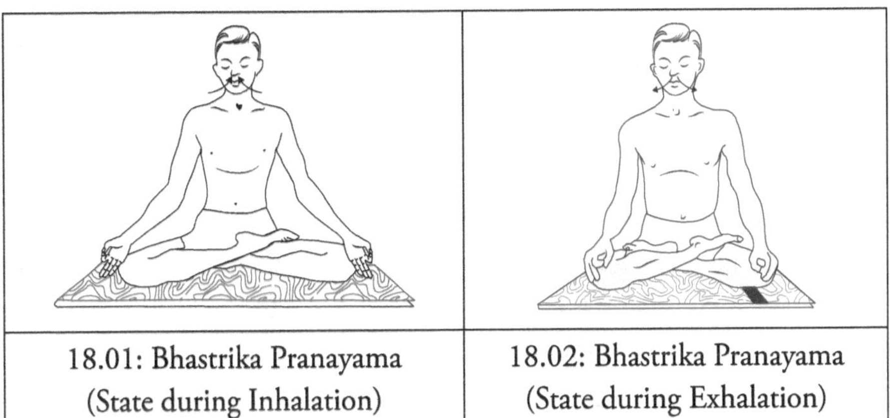

18.01: Bhastrika Pranayama (State during Inhalation)	18.02: Bhastrika Pranayama (State during Exhalation)

- This Pranayama can be practised in three stages according to one's own capacity, i.e., **slow, medium and fast**. Those with weak lungs and heart should go slow by inhaling and exhaling slowly. Exhalations should be soft and smooth. A healthy and old practitioner may gradually proceed with the process at medium pace and then fast. It may be practised for three to five minutes.

- In this Pranayama, while inhaling breath, one should fill his mind with the thought that the all-pervading cosmic power and the celestial energy, peace, tranquillity, bliss, purity of oxygen and whatever else is pure and chaste is pouring into me with breath. I am being engulfed by the externally available cosmic power.

Kapalabhati Pranayama

This is the king of all Pranayama techniques. 'Kapala' means brain and 'Bhati' means to shine (Enlightenment of the intellect). The process which leads to enhance the shining of the face and mind is called 'Kapalabhati' Pranayama.

Technique:

In terms of techniques, it only slightly varies from the process of 'Bhastrika' Pranayama. In 'Bhastrika' Pranayama, equal force is applied on inhaling and exhaling, whereas, in 'Kapalabhati,' maximum pressure is applied on exhaling the breath. An effort to inhale is not forcefully done but it is allowed to occur in a normal, natural and instinctive way. Full concentration is applied to exhaling of the breath. In this Pranayama, deflation and inflation of the belly takes place automatically.

Each exhalation is to be performed in synchronised manner. Each exhalation should involve all body organs as elaborated. Hips – should experience mild contraction. Pelvic region – should experience mild upward thrust. Belly – should be pressed inwards with each exhalation. Spine and wind/food pipe – must be erect, stretched upward, still with no movements. Nostrils – should be expanding for exhaling and inhaling in natural manner. Eyes – Closed. Mind – Focussed.

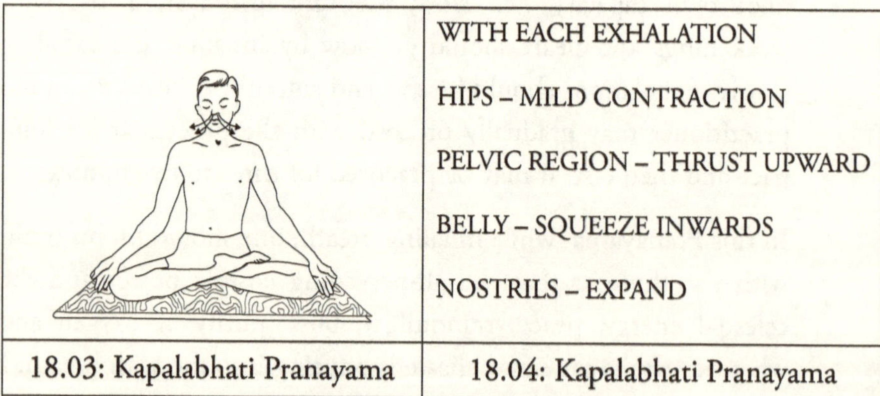

18.03: Kapalabhati Pranayama	18.04: Kapalabhati Pranayama

Initially to get acquainted with the practice and before understanding the finer nuances, start with twenty to twenty-five breaths (forceful exhalations) per minute first and then increase practice. Normally thirty to thirty-five breaths per minute is a good speed.

While doing 'Kapalabhati' Pranayama, one should think that all ailments of one's mind and body are exiting with each exhalation and are getting destroyed. Exhaling should be with the thought that I am releasing all my physical diseases and mental ailments. This will generate positive thoughts in the mind throughout. This Pranayama can also be performed in three variants, slow, medium and fast.

Slow: Frequency of exhalations should be roughly one per second, translating into, fifty-five to sixty-five exhalations per minute. Breathing out is silent, without producing any audible sound. All organs are however involved as explained above. This is of meditative nature and is beneficial for mind.

Medium: Frequency of exhalation is thirty to forty per minute. Exhalation sound is normally audible, without consciously making sound. All organs are involved as explained before. This has mild cleansing effect on wind pipe, vocal folds and mind.

Fast: Breathing out is forced, with full energy, as in 'Bhastrika' Pranayama. Frequency twenty to thirty breaths per minute. Sound of expelled air shall be easily audible. This has an effect of cleansing the complete respiratory system.

Once you start practising this exercise, remember, I strongly recommended it. You are likely to encounter a dilemma about the correct speed and intensity. The intensity of the 'Kapalabhati' can be better understood with knowledge of its primary benefits. It is an effort at cleaning your respiratory system and mind. The efforts of cleaning are required to be commensurate with the expected dust and dirt deposits on these organs. You are in best position to judge the quantity and quality of these deposits.

So, you may accordingly decide on speed, intensity and the time span to be allocated to this exercise.

If you are doing it initially or after significant time gaps, with your system carrying a huge baggage of your inverted lifestyles, make it as intense as feasible. For a regular practitioner, a slow version for three to five minutes is good enough. For best results in routine practices, remember my section on "Storytelling and Yoga." One may start with slow (for one to two minutes), progress to mild (for one to two minutes), reach peak (maximum one minute) and finally end with slow (say one to two minutes)

Try out the following fun activities also, while performing 'Kapalabhati':

1. While performing 'Kapalabhati,' shift the focus of your attention from one organ to another. Starting from left and right hemispheres of brain, traverse downwards. Involving all important organs of mind, forehead, head, eyes, ears, cheeks, dentures, neck, heart, lungs, kidney etc. etc., build a thought in your mind that the impurities, the stress, the dust and dirt deposited on that organ, are being expelled through breath. Perform five to ten exhalations for each important organ. Involve as many internal and external organs as you can.

2. You may also add an element of tapping or massaging, pressing (e.g., stretch your eyelids slightly downwards, building a mild pressure on eye-socket), or stretching (e.g., catch holds of your ears with both hands and push the earlobes downwards with hands straight and hands crossed, sideways, and upwards) on that specific organ. Thus, while exhaling, keeping in mind a specific organ, say ears, pull the earlobes downwards, sideways and upwards. Similarly, massage gently the heart region, while performing 'kapalabhati' with heart prominently placed in mind.

Anuloma-Viloma Pranayama

The main feature of this Pranayama is alternate breathing through the left and the right nostrils, without or with retention of breath ('Kumbhaka'). 'Viloma' means produced in the reverse order. This Pranayama gets its name from the fact that the order of breathing through the nostrils for inhalation and exhalation is reversed every time.

Techniques:

1. For ease of focus and concentration, place the tip of index finger of right hand over the focal point, maintaining mild pressure on focal point. Create an inverted tong kind of formation, with your right hand. Tip of index finger placed on focal point, is to act as the topmost fixed point, where the tong is firmly hung downwards. One arm of this tong is right thumb, which is to be used for closing and opening the right nostril. The other arm is the second finger, which is to be used for opening and closing the left nostril. Now close the right nostril with the right thumb, and inhale through the left open nostril, right thumb remaining on and closing tightly the right nostril (See 18.05).

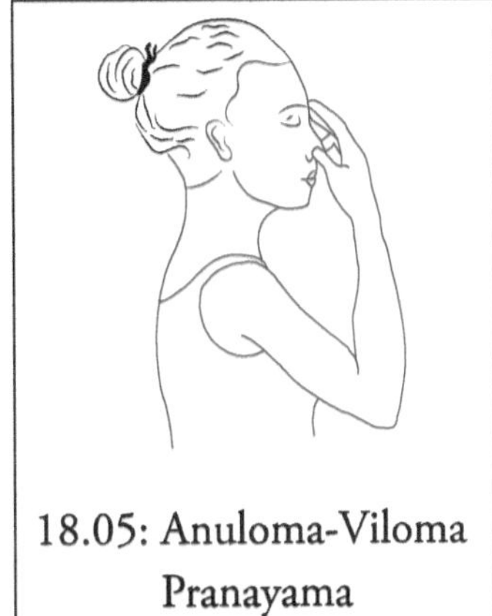

18.05: Anuloma-Viloma Pranayama

2. Now release the right nostril and close the left nostril with the index finger of right hand and exhale normally, with no undue force, through the right nostril.

3. Holding the left nostril still closed as above, inhale through the right nostril (See 18.06). Now release the left nostril and close the right nostril with the right thumb as in (See 18.05) above, but exhale through the left nostril, and still holding the right nostril

with the right thumb, inhale through the left nostril as in (1) above This is one round. You may start with five to ten rounds and practise this Pranayama for about three to five minutes.

Pranayama is a process of regulation of the breath resulting in silencing the mind. Even a few rounds of Pranayama of moderate measure properly practised should give you an experience of peace of mind. Even without my prodding, you should be able to conclude that this Pranayama helps you in maintaining the right-left balance of your breathing and bodily functions.

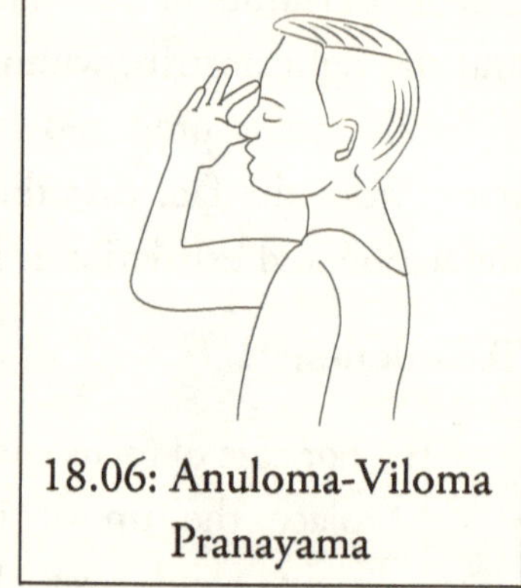

18.06: Anuloma-Viloma Pranayama

Anuloma-Viloma can also be practised with three variations as under:

Mild: In this version, both inhalation and exhalation are performed slowly and gently, without exerting any extra pressure or applying extra energy for both actions. You may maintain a good speed here and keep on shifting the thumb from one nostril to finger on another on a faster pace. Keep the inhalation, retention and exhalation times as equals.

Moderate: In this, both 'Uddiyan Bandha' and 'Moola Bandha' are applied to forcefully increase the volume of sucked in air during inhalation. Retention ('Kumbhak') is normal. Exhalation is performed at normal pace after sequentially releasing first 'Uddiyan Bandha' and thereafter 'Moola Bandha.' Speed is normally half of mild version one.

Intense: Here in addition to the 'Uddiyan' Bandha and 'Moola' Bandha in inhalation, 'Jalandhar' Bandha is also applied in retention phase ('Kumbhaka'). The steps are: (1) **Inhale:** Right nostril, left closed, apply 'Moola' Bandha, apply 'Uddiyan' Bandha. (2) **Retain:** Close both nostrils, apply 'Jalandhar' Bandha. (3) **Exhale:** Release 'Jalandhar' Bandha. Open left nostril, release 'Uddiyan' Bandha, release 'Moola' Bandha, exhale. (4) **Inhale:** Left nostril, right closed, apply 'Moola' Bandha, apply

'Uddiyan' Bandha. (5) **Retain:** Close both nostrils, apply 'Jalandhar' Bandha. (6) **Exhale:** Release 'Jalandhar' Bandha, open right nostril, release 'Uddiyan' Bandha, release 'Moola' Bandha, exhale. This completes one round.

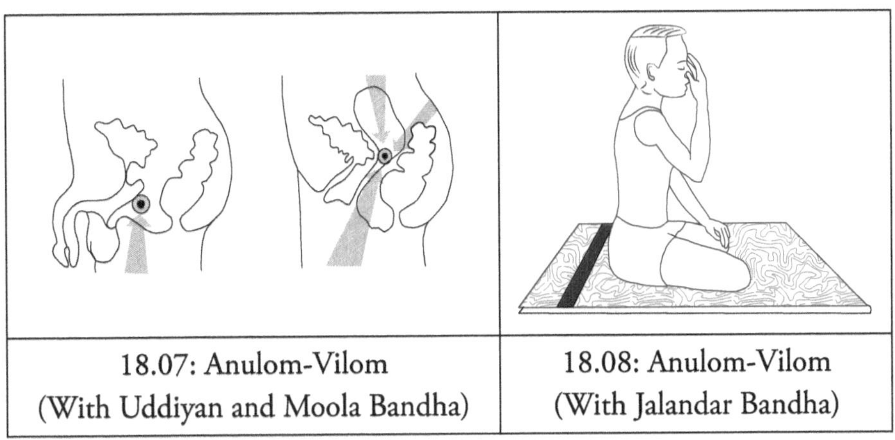

18.07: Anulom-Vilom (With Uddiyan and Moola Bandha)	18.08: Anulom-Vilom (With Jalandar Bandha)

Benefits:

The main purpose of this Pranayama is to purify the principal channels carrying energy called Nadi's. Hence it nourishes the whole body, induces tranquillity and helps to improve concentration. It increases vitality and lowers the level of stress and anxiety. It cures cough disorders. It is also effective in ensuring that both nostrils share equal burden of breathing process.

If you can perform all three variants of these three pranayamas, half of the battle of acquiring knowledge on Pranayama is already won.

Day-Nineteen: Easy, Effective, Everyday Pranayama: Part – II

Learning and Practice for the Day

Today we will continue learning some more of easy practices useful for day-to-day practising of 'Pranayama.'

Bhramari Pranayama

Have you ever minutely observed the life of a honeybee? It is so sweet (honey), so colourful (flowers) and so musical (humming all the time). We may experience one-third of the joys of life of a honey bee by humming like it. Humming like a bee is Bhramari Pranayama. The name is derived from 'Bhramara' (a black bee).

Precautions:

To be avoided in case of nose and ear infections. Not to be overdone as this Pranayama involves working on some very sensitive glands in your body.

Techniques:

Sit on 'Padmasana' or 'Siddhasana.' For facilitating concentration and focus, close both ears by inserting respective thumbs in cavities of ears. Close left ear with left thumb and right ear with right thumb. Allow all fingers to envelop your face, let the tips of index fingers be pointing towards the focal point. Keep the eyes closed; if considered necessary, you may place one or two fingers on the eyelids to ensure forced closure of eyes.

This body posture is also called 'Sunmukhi Mudra.' (See 19.01) Now inhale rapidly through both nostrils making sound of 'Bhramara,' the bee, and exhale rapidly through both nostrils, making the humming sound. The desired tonal quality of sound here is the same as the last variation of the sound in 'AUM' recitations to pronounce 'MMM… MMM.' One deep inhalation and one exhalation accompanied with prolonged humming sound

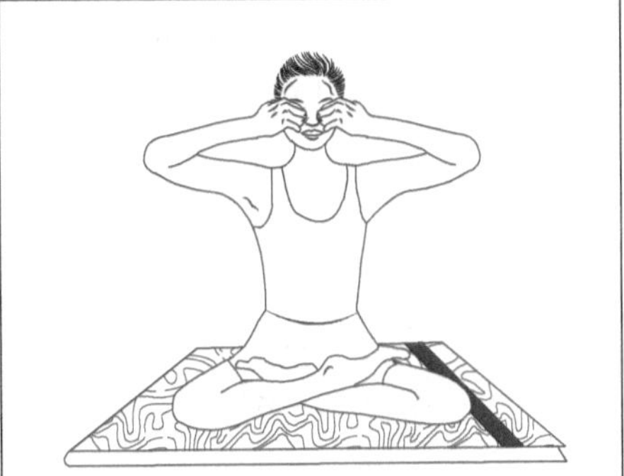

19.01: Bhramari Pranayama
(Sunmukhi Mudra)

complete one round. You can carry the process till the body is bathed in perspiration. In the end, inhale through both nostrils, retain the breath for as long as you can do it comfortably and then exhale slowly through both nostrils.

It is stated in literatures, that the joy which the practitioner gets in making the 'Kumbhaka' during Bhramari Pranayama is unlimited and indescribable. In the beginning, heat of the body is increased as the circulation of blood is quickened. In the end the body heat is decreased by perspiration. By success in this 'Bhramari Kumbhaka,' the Yogic student gets success in Samadhi.

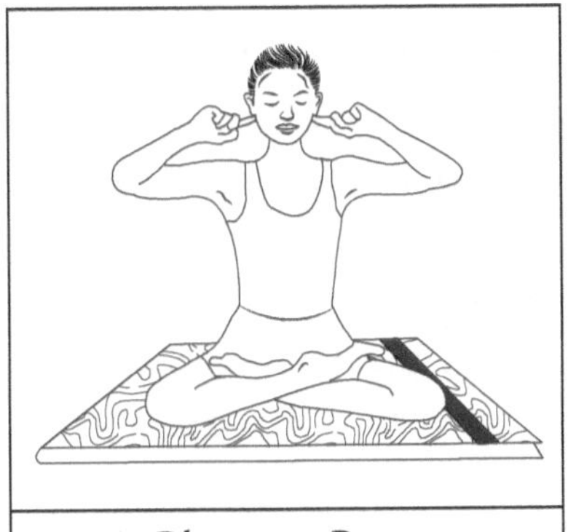

19.02: Bhramari Pranayama

The suggested actions of forcibly closing the eyes and ears are applicable only for beginners. Once you attain reasonable proficiency, it is advisable to keep hands free, placed comfortably on knees, fingers forming 'Jnana' or 'Chin' Mudra. The inhalation, exhalation and humming actions remain the same. (See 19.02).

Benefits:

The practice of this Pranayama relieves stress and helps in alleviating anxiety, anger and hyper-activity.

The resonance effect of humming sound creates a soothing effect on the mind and nervous system.

It is a great tranquiliser found good in the management of stress related disorders. It is a useful preparatory Pranayama for concentration and meditation.

A word of caution: This practice is so soothing and enjoyable, that it is almost addictive. Once you start enjoying it, you may not feel like migrating to other exercises/Asanas. You may tend to overdo it. This Pranayama works on a few of the very sensitive glands in your body. Overdoing is not recommended; it may make those glands hyperactive, which is not desirable and may cause some moderate harm. It is best to practice it on alternate days only, i.e., three to four times in a week during routine practices. Average recommended repetitions are five in numbers.

You may also try some more fun and variations while practising Bhramari Pranayama.

1. Try to place the upper teeth line just above the lower teeth line, keeping fractions of millimetres gap between upper and lower teeth lines, so that the vibrations caused by the humming sound of breathing cause vibrations and variations in gaps between teeth. You should experience some mild, good, funny and enjoyable, chattering sound and vibrations in jaw-lines. It may be difficult to achieve initially as precision is required in maintaining the gap and amount of pressure between teeth. But the results are very sweet. Try it! The resultant experience will be worth the efforts.

2. While sitting in 'Sunmukhi' Mudra and humming out during exhalations, try to alternatively release and press again, the thumbs in the ear cavities. This should bring in a musical variation in

the sound of humming that you are hearing. The experience is musically good.

Mahabandha Pranayama (With the Three Bandhas)

These pranayamas are breath holding exercises, with application of all three 'Bandhas,' i.e., Jalandhar Bandha, Uddiyan Bandha and Moolabandha. There are two variations depending upon application of Bandha after inhalation or after exhalation as under:

Techniques:

A. Bahya Mahabandha:

Sitting in anyone posture, either Vajrasana, Siddhasana or in Padmasana, exhale to capacity, with a forceful exhalation as in Bhastrika Pranayama.

Hold the breath out and apply all the three Bandhas. Follow the sequence of 'Uddiyan' Bandha first, followed by 'Moola' Bandha and finally the 'Jalandhar' Bandha. When there is a need to take breath, first remove the three Bandhas smoothly and sequentially, and breathe in slowly. Repeat this process for three to twenty-one times.

This is called Bahya (External) Mahabandha Pranayama.

B. Antrik Mahabandha:

Sit in any meditative posture and take a long breath in, hold and apply the three Bandhas as in 'Bahya Mahabandha' in smooth and sequential manner.

The only difference between 'Bahya' and 'Antrik Mahabandha' is that in the former we exhale, hold and then apply the three Bandhas, while in 'Antrik Mahabandha,' we inhale, hold and then apply the three Bandhas (Mahabandha).

This Pranayama is complimentary to 'Bahya Mahabandha,' i.e., after performing one round of 'Bahya Mahabandha,' perform one round of

'Antrik Mahabandha.' One round of 'Antrik Mahabandha' followed by one round of 'Bahya Mahabandha' makes one round of 'Mahabandha' Pranayama.

Benefits: In this Pranayama also, like 'Kapalabhati' all negative thoughts are pushed out while exhaling. All problems and ailments will be over to the extent of one's determination and resolute thinking. The divine/creative thoughts in the mind are considered to be the annihilator of any kind of physical and mental diseases and negativities.

Day-Twenty: Some More Pranayama Exercises

Learning for the Day

The fun breathing exercises, during the initial learning phase, and the five pranayamas termed as 'Easy, Effective, Everyday Pranayama' with their variants learnt so far, are adequate to meet your requirements of remaining happy and healthy, while living your everyday life. Even after you adopt Yoga in your life and start practising daily, you will find it difficult to squeeze in all the 'Pranayama' exercises in your daily routine. Each exercise has two to three variants and versions. So, you have effectively learnt ten to fifteen different Pranayama exercises.

No matter howsoever sincere you are in you endeavours to adopt Yoga and practise daily routines, monotony invariably brings in boredom. If you decide upon one package, involving three to four Pranayamas to be practised daily, sooner or later your interest will start declining. To safeguard against these monotonies, boredoms, and disinterests, it should make sense to keep on varying your package. The learning of today is therefore important. We are going to learn a few more of Pranayama exercises today. You may add one or more of these pranayamas to your base pack crafted out of your learnings from Day-sixteen to Day-nineteen for some variations, sparks and sparkles.

Pranayama and Meditation

Pranayama occurs naturally during meditation. When you concentrate during meditation, the breath automatically becomes slower and slower.

You actually experience this meditative Pranayama daily unconsciously. When you read an interesting fiction or a sensational storybook or when you are engrossed in solving a complex mathematical problem, crosswords or puzzle, your mind gets fully absorbed in the subject matter.

If you closely observe your breath on these occasions, you will find that the breath has become very, very slow. Slow breathings help you in concentration and focus. The reverse of this is also true. Similarly, when you see a tragic story being enacted in the theatre or a film show, or when you hear a very sad piece of news or some joyful, elating news, or when you shed tears either of joy or sorrow, or burst into laughter, the breath gets slackened. Thus, Pranayama occurs by itself.

It is obvious from these examples, that when the mind is deeply concentrated on any subject, the respiration slows down or stops. Pranayama is thus occurring automatically. Mind and breath are intimately and intricately connected. If you turn your attention to observantly watch the breath on those occasions, it will soon regain its normal and natural pace.

Pranayama and Walking

If walking is your current form of favourite exercise or your passion, you may add some more value to it, by performing Pranayama during walking. Always walk with head held high, shoulders back and with chest expanded. Inhale slowly through both nostrils, keep counting and chanting 'AUM or OHM' (if comfortable with the word, sound and symbols, else you may choose similar word for slow rhythmic and smooth chant) mentally synchronising your chanting with your steps. It shall be best, if you can select a long, straight obstruction-free stretch of path for practising Pranayama during walking. Select any pointed object, in the line of vision at the end of the path/road stretch, or in the horizon and fix your gaze at this point. Now walk with gaze fixed at one point, spine and head straight, while chanting 'AUM.' Try to achieve a pace of one count/one chant for each step. If it is initially difficult to match speeds of chanting and stepping, try to build synchronisation in some other format, i.e., one chant for three steps or two steps for one chant.

When tired and taking small breaks or relaxing during walking, relax by retaining the breath till you count 'AUM or OHM' for minimum twelve times (i.e., breathing in four times and chanting 'Aum' three times after each breathing in). You may make a circular 360-degree rotation, chanting longer version of 'OHM' three times for each direction, i.e., facing north, chant three times, then turn east, chant three times and so on. Keep a positive thought in mind, while facing each direction, that you are drawing energy or purity available in that direction for yourself. Thereafter, exhale slowly through both nostrils till you count 'AUM' or 'OHM' twelve times. Take the respiratory pause or rest after one Pranayama, i.e., after walking one stretch. If you find it difficult to synchronise 'AUM' chanting with steps, you may chant AUM without linking it with the steps.

'Kapalabhati' can also be performed during walking. If you are very busy and are unable to allocate separate time for Yoga, you may practise 'Kapalabhati' Pranayama during your morning or evening walks. It will give you twin advantages of Pranayama as well as of walking. You will find it very pleasant to practise Pranayama while walking in an open place, when delightful gentle breeze is blowing, and fresh oxygen-rich air is in abundance. You will be invigorated and rejuvenated quickly to a considerable degree. Practise, feel and realise the marked, beneficial influence of this kind of Pranayama. Those who walk briskly, either repeating OHM mentally or verbally or keeping focus on breathings, do practise natural Pranayama without any effort.

For performing 'Kapalabhati' during walking also, fix your vision at one fixed point in the horizon, walk while exhaling only, synchronising one exhalation for one step. Initially, it may be difficult to synchronise exhalations with steps. Start with forcefully exhaling while walking and slowly develop the habit of matching speed of steps with breathing.

Pranayama, Meditation and Shavasana

We had earlier dealt with the issues of meditation and Shavasana. We have already discussed that Shavasana is the best Asana for meditation, except for the problem of tendencies to drift away to sleep, while in Shavasana. Let us now experience all the three together, i.e., Pranayama, meditation and Shavasana. Lie down on the back, quite at ease, over a blanket/mat. Keep the hands on the ground by the side, about six inches away from body, and legs straight. The heels should be kept together, but the toes can remain a little apart. Relax all the muscles and the nerves. Those who are physically very weak or suffering from problems of pains in lower back, can practise Pranayama in this pose while lying on the ground or on a bed sheet.

Draw the breath slowly without making any noise, through both nostrils (remember, not through mouth as is normally done in Shavasana for quicker relaxation). Retain the breath, if you can do it with comfort. Then exhale slowly through both nostrils. You may repeat this process twelve to twenty-one times in the morning and in the evening. Chant 'OHM' mentally (if comfortable with the word, sound and symbols, else may choose similar word for slow rhythmic and smooth chant) during the practice.

This is a combined exercise of asana, Pranayama, meditation and rest. It gives rest not only to the body but also to the mind. It gives relief, comfort and ease. This is suitable for aged people. Be watchful and guard against the tendency of falling asleep. Better perform in group or in the presence of family members.

Surya Bheda Pranayama

Sit on 'Sukhasana,' 'Ardhpadmasana,' 'Padmasana' or 'Siddhasana.' Close the eyes. Keep the left nostril closed, with your right ring and little fingers applying moderate pressures. Slowly inhale, without making any audible sound, for as long as you can do it comfortably, through the right nostril. Then, close the right nostril with your right thumb and retain the breath, firmly pressing the chin against the chest (i.e., apply 'Jalandhar Bandha').

Hold on to the breath till tired to the extent that perspiration oozes from the tips of the nails and roots of the hairs (hair follicles). This point cannot be reached easily by the beginners during the initial practices.

One needs to increase the period of 'Kumbhaka' gradually to enable perfection. This is considered to be the limit of the sphere of practice of 'Surya Bheda Kumbhaka.' Then exhale very slowly, without making any audible sound, through the left nostril by closing the right nostril with the thumb. Chant 'OHM' mentally with feelings and appreciating the meanings during inhalation, retention and exhalation. Exhale after purifying the skull by forcing the breath consciously upwards.

This Pranayama should be repeatedly performed, as it purifies the brain and destroys the intestinal worms and diseases arising from excess of abdominal wind.

Ujjayi Pranayama

Sit comfortably in any of 'Sukhasana,' 'Ardhpadmasana,' 'Padmasana' or 'Siddhasana' posture. Close the mouth. Inhale slowly through both the nostrils in a smooth, uniform manner till the breath fills the space from the throat to the heart. Retain the breath for as long as you can comfortably do it and then exhale slowly through the left nostril by closing the right nostril with your right thumb.

Expand the chest when you inhale. During inhalation a peculiar sound is produced owing to the partial closing of glottis. The sound produced during inhalation should be of a mild and uniform pitch. It should be continuous also. This 'Kumbhaka' may be practised even when walking or standing. Instead of exhaling through the left nostril, you can exhale slowly through both nostrils.

Sitkari Pranayama

Sit comfortably in any of meditation postures, i.e., 'Sukhasana,' 'Ardhpadmasana,' 'Padmasana,' 'Vajrasana' or 'Siddhasana.' Fold the tongue, in circular manner upwards and then in backwards direction, so that the tip of the tongue might touch the upper palate.

Then draw the air through the mouth with a hissing sound "C...... C...... C...... C" (or Si, Si, Si, Si). There after retain the breath for as long as you can do without feeling suffocated and then exhale slowly through both nostrils.

You can keep the two rows of teeth in contact with each other and then inhale the air through the mouth as before.

Sitali Pranayama

Sit comfortably in any of meditation postures, i.e., 'Sukhasana,' 'Ardhpadmasana,' 'Padmasana' or 'Siddhasana.' Protrude the tongue outwards a little far away from the lips. Fold the tongue to give it a shape resembling a tube.

Draw in the air through the mouth with the hissing sound "Si." Retain the breath for as long as you can hold on with comfort. Then exhale slowly through both nostrils. Practise this daily again and again in the morning from fifteen to thirty times.

You can do this sitting in any variant of 'Vajrasana' or even when you are standing or walking. However, take care; your whistling sound should not land you in trouble and accusations of 'eve-teasing.'

Day Twenty-One: Packaged Stress Busters: Part – I

Learning for the Day

Stress is the most common subject of discussion in the context of Yoga. It is referred to and associated with everything from occasional mild irritations to acute depression. Do you think I am novice enough to unnecessarily take on the stress of defining stress? You all know what stress is. You also know its effect on our health, happiness and wellbeing. This menace is increasing exponentially with each change of generation.

I am presenting here a few packages to take care of your stresses. Your learning and acceptances may get enhanced, if you know the science behind them. The packages basically incorporate the bests of following:

Meditation

Meditation is the best antidote to stress. If you know good meditation practices, can devote fifteen to twenty minutes every day and are able to effectively meditate, you have already achieved immunity to stress. You need not bother about my packages. However, regular, effective meditation, particularly for intellectuals, atheists, professionals, rationalists, and those obsessed with science, is a utopian dream. Controlling hyper-activity of mind for such persons is very difficult. Hence the attractively packaged stress busters are needed.

Breathing

Breathing, particularly the slow repeated exhalations, as in 'Kapalabhati,' have an immense positive influence on your brain. An excellent way to relieve stress in a few minutes, it is much faster than cooking instant noodles.

Clapping

We clap when we feel good. When we see some live performance, a song, dance, poetry-recitation, a good intelligent punch in a comic performance, a powerful dialogue in a theatrical event, or a good satire, we automatically feel the urge to appreciate.

We clap to express our appreciation automatically. Clapping is seldom forced. You only intentionally force your clapping when the performer is your spouse or your boss. After all, you need to live for the next day. In normal circumstances, it is a natural, instinctive, automatic, spontaneous reaction of feeling good, feeling happy, and an evocation of the urge to smile or laugh.

For clapping to physically happen, the sensors, the receptors in your sensory organs need to sense some presence of hormones, chemicals, DNA, genome or whatsoever else is required for these sensors to generate a signal to the brain. The signal is transmitted in real time, to your own supercomputer, your brain. Your brain processes this signal. If appreciation is approved, brain transmits signal to your hands utilising nerves, electrical pulses in Nano-Volts and Nano-Ampere range to clap. Your hands clap utilising power through muscles.

So, it is not only your hands that appreciate, it is you, your body, your brain, all get involved in the process of appreciation, feeling good, happy, or humorous.

For every action, there is an equal and opposite reaction. It is the law of nature. It must follow, that we may generate the same hormones, genome, or DNA associated with the feelings of happiness, wellbeing, appreciation, smiles and laughter by application of laws of science. If urge to laugh provokes clapping, clapping should also provoke urge to laugh. If smile on the face provokes clapping, clapping should also bring smile on the face.

It happens that we can confuse our body, confuse ourselves, and evoke the same emotions, the same pleasures, as in an exceptionally good live performance. So, clap, clap and clap! If you find my explanation of the benefits of clapping to be good, you may convey your appreciation by a good round of applause. Clap firmly! Clap to make some noise! Clap to stir some air! Clap to appreciate others! Clap for no reasons! Clap for your own good!

Positive-Auto-Suggestions

I need not over emphasize the benefits of these in relieving stress. Your mind will feel what you ask it to feel. It may not listen to you at once. It may not respond to your first call. But when you repeatedly and consistently ask it to do something, it cannot remain immune to your commands and your pleadings. It will succumb to the pressure. After all, it is your brain, your mind.

Acupressure and Acupuncture

These are proven branches of medical sciences.

Talking to Your Body Organs

You may not believe it. You may initially not accept that you can actually talk to organs in your body, your lungs, your heart, your pancreas, your thyroid glands, your legs, arms, eyes, ears, nose and so on. The statement that these organs listen to your commands, follow them, and report and talk-back to you, may not be very palatable, unless you really experience it. Follow the instructions blindly, having faith. First try it; believe it thereafter. Just leave your inhibitions, set aside your reservations and follow the commands. Assume that you have adopted me as your 'Guru.'

Laughter Therapy

Laughter, as you know, is not a mere gesture of your facial muscles for expressions of fun. It is universally acknowledged as a therapy for many diseases and ailments, stress related disorders, being the prime ones.

Package Number 1

Steps:

1. Follow the prerequisites! You know what they are!

2. Sit in any comfortable meditation posture, 'Sukhasana,' 'Padmasana,' 'Vajrasana,' or on chair. Keep body and arms loose and relaxed, spine straight, head high, eyes closed, ears selectively receptive to pleasing sounds only, hands resting on your knees, hanging loosely on your arms, fingers forming Jnana or Chin Mudra. Sit at ease, enjoying, mind focussed on focal point. Install image of Guru or creator in your mind.

3. Cross check all your body parts. See that there is no undue stretching, undue tension or pressure. Loosen everything. If you find some mild pain, tension, stretching, talk to the organ to loosen up and to relax.

4. Take a deep breath, and chant 'OHM' as explained in Chapter-One Day-twelve.

5. Now fold your hands in front of your face, joining both palms together, keeping hands just a few millimetres away from the tip of your nose. This is Namaste posture. (Namaskar Mudra). Relax in this posture; count your breaths by counting to thirty.

6. Say your prayers. Spend at least one minute on your prayers.

7. Now clap your hands vigorously, with as much force as you can comfortably tolerate. Take hands as apart as feasible, clap in front of your face, each clap culminating just a few millimetres away from the tip of your nose. Feel the air expelled from the force of your clapping on your face, in your eyes, on your nose. Count the clap sounds.

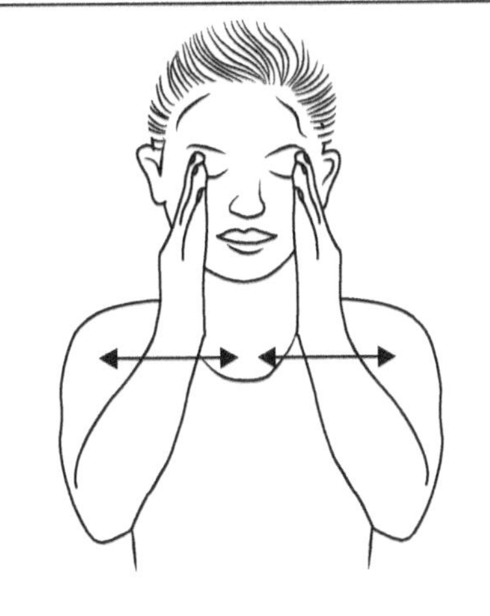

21.01: Clapping

8. Feel the rush of extra blood onto your palms. Enjoy the reddening of your palms.

9. Ensure no jerky movements. Each clap should be as smoothly flowing as water flows, and in dance-like movements.

10. Count at least 121 claps or two minutes of clapping.

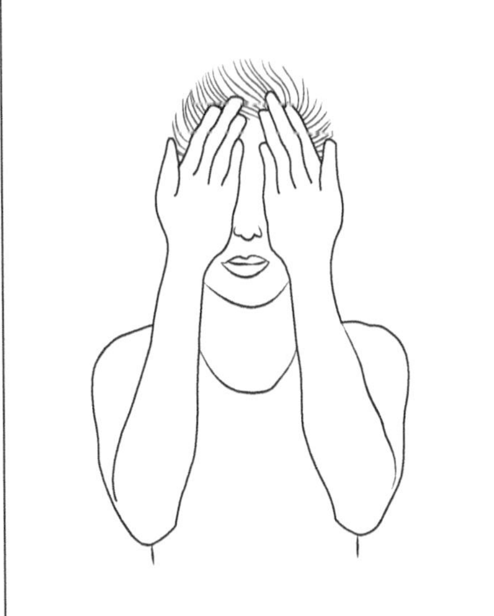

21.02: Palming the Eyes

11. Now put your hand on your face, bottom portion of the palms firmly resting on your closed eyelids, palms gently pressing the eyelids, filling up the full socket of your eyes. Fingers should be pointing upwards, covering your forehead, and gently bent in a curve to match the profile of your forehead. Tips of the fingers should gently press the centre line of your head, the central parting line of your hair.

12. Feel the heat transfer to your eyes, the retina, and through your eyes to your face.

13. Some of the static electricity generated is also being discharged, and dissipated to your face through your eyes and forehead.

14. Relax. Relax and Relax in this posture, till your palms feels normal, reach the normal temperature, and extra reddening disappears. This should normally take thirty to forty-five seconds.

15. Now we will massage our face and head as is done in facials in make-up. Massage your face and head with palms and fingers. While moving smoothly on your face, the palms should follow profile of the face always maintaining the gentle pressure. Massage your face ten times with right hand moving in anti-clockwise direction and left hand encircling the face in clockwise direction. When hands are traversing upwards, fingers should cover the skull. Count each rotation. Count ten.

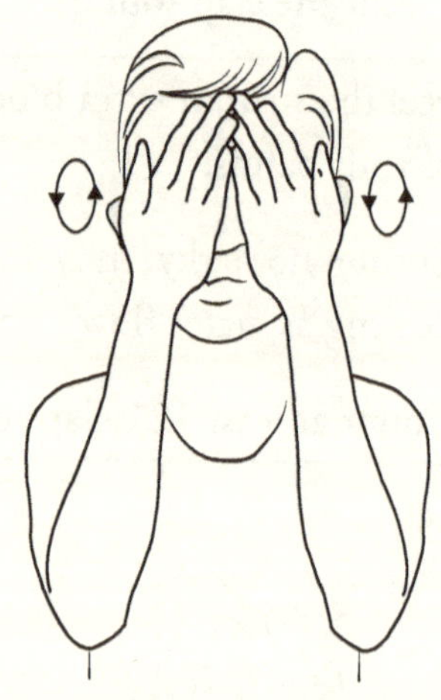

21.03: Face Massage

16. Now repeat the face massage in opposite directions. Right hand moving in clockwise directions and left hand moving in anti-clock wise direction. Count ten.

17. Relax! Relax! And Relax!

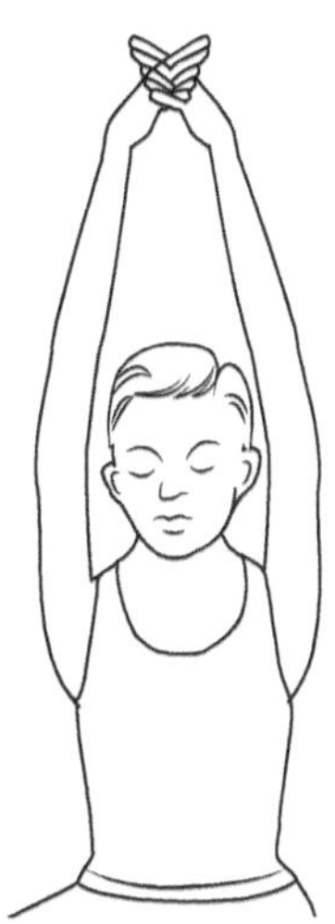

21.04: Hands Raised and Joined

18. Now gently take both your hands vertically up above your head making a smooth curvature like movement. Join both hands together, your arms forming an inverted 'V' formation. Now form an X formation with your thumbs and fingers by inserting fingers of right hand in gaps between fingers of left hand, keeping your left thumb over right thumb. Now form a tight fist with both palms. See the picture 21.04.

19. Stretch your full body upwards gently but firmly. Relax.

20. Now move your hands downwards retaining the fist-formation and place your palms in locked position at the neck. Your hands should press your neck forward hard and neck should apply equal pressure on your hands and push them backwards, such that no appreciable movement take place. Retain this posture for five to ten seconds. (See 21.05)

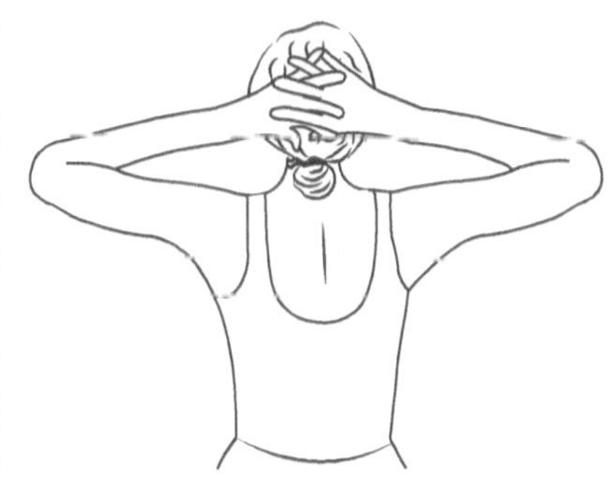

21.05: Neck Pressing

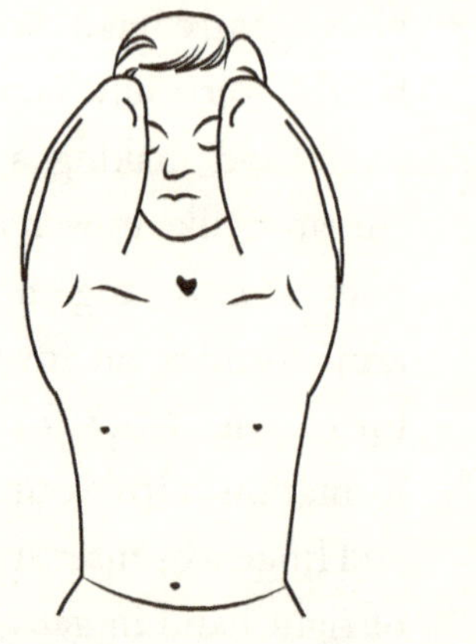

21.06: Pressing Neck with Arms

21. Now remaining in this position, bring both your arms in front with your palms firmly holding the neck. Try to push both arms such that elbow bone of right hand touches the elbow bone of left hand. Hold and release. Take both arms in front, palms placed on your neck firmly gripping the neck. (See 21.06)

22. Repeat Step 21 five to ten times.

23. Now keeping your fingers locked, hand fist intact, take both hands above your head and make one firm upward stretch and release the fist. Sit comfortably and relax.

24. Bend your right hand and bring your hand in front of your chest, palm facing away from your face. Bend your fingers slightly towards left to form shape of English alphabet "U." (See 21.07)

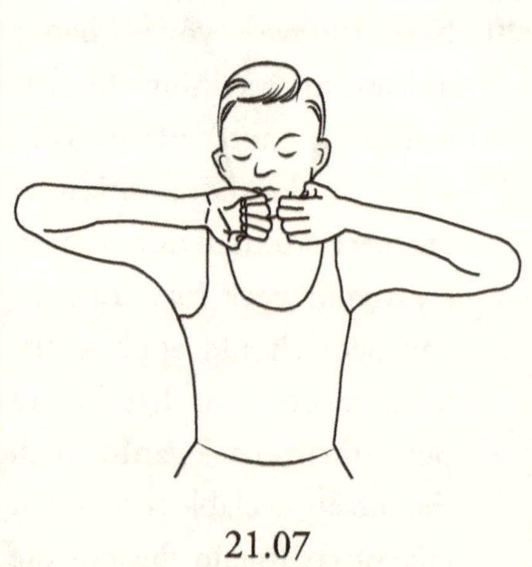

21.07

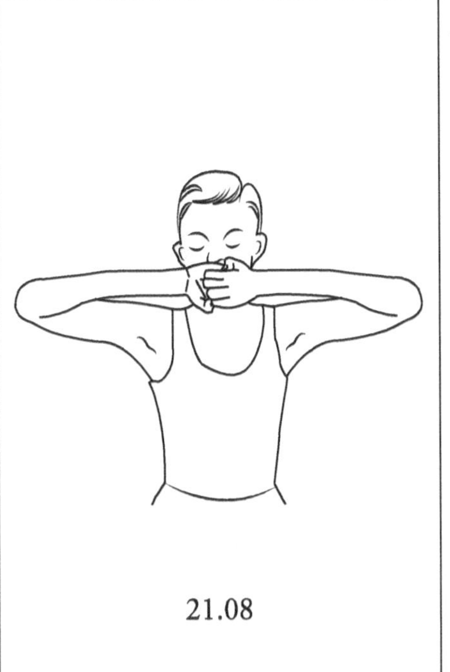

21.08

25. Bring your left hand also in front of your chest, with palm facing towards your face. Make a "U" formation with your fingers. Interlock both hands by inserting left hand's "U" formed fingers into the cavity of right hand "U" formed fingers. Stretch your left arm leftwards and right arm rightward such that the "U" interlocked fingers feel good amount of pressure. Release the stretching of arms, retaining the hands locked at fingers-end and "U" formed locked fingers. (See 21.08).

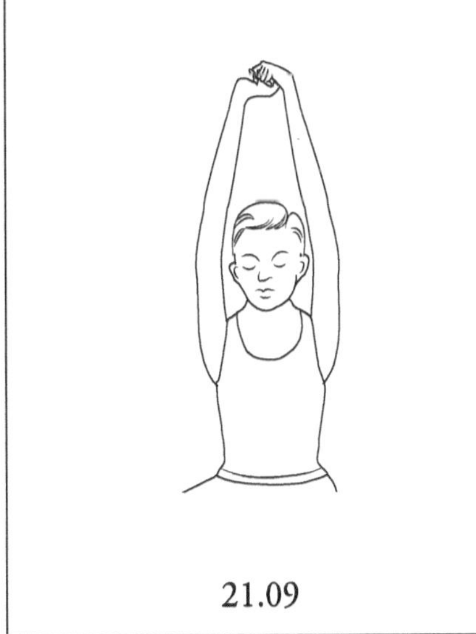

21.09

26. Take both hands upwards over your head retaining the hands grip. Allow hands to be slightly backwards, giving your upper body a slight backwards push. Keep head firm and vertical. (See 21.09).

27. Now bring your right arm downwards, keeping left arm up, such that the interlocked gripped fist touches at side of your neck and just below your head on the backside. Stretch your left arm upwards, and right arm downwards, the interlocked fingers feeling the pressure. Your hands should apply force on your head and neck trying to push it forward. Your neck and head should apply equal pressure in opposite directions to maintain balance, head retaining its position and refusing to move. Hold for a few seconds and thereafter release. (See 21.10).

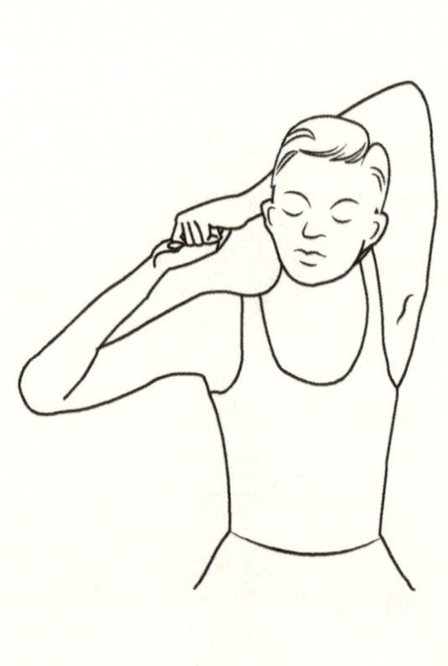

21.10

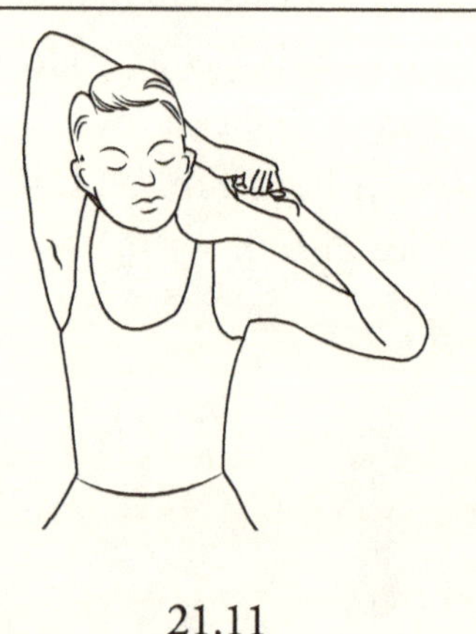

21.11

28. Now repeat Step 27 with your right arm going up, left arm coming down, fist with fingers interlocked pushing your head and neck joint as before. Repeat Step 27 and 28 five to ten times. (See 21.11)

29. Relax! Relax! and Relax.

30. Take a deep breath and make a loud recitation of "Aum" or "Ohm."

Package Number 2

The highlights of this package are, while performing 'Kapalabhati, (slow, relaxed, and meditative exhalations, at pace of one per second, with no audible breathing sounds) focussing your mind on all important internal organs and external body parts, and mentally talking to organs/body parts, covering your body from head to toe and toe to head, internally and externally.

You must make a conscious effort to focus your attention, your mind on the organ/part and say a few positive sentences to each part. You may thank, appreciate, and praise them. You may form your own conversation, your own paragraphs and set of sentences for each organ. Just to lead you on the path, some illustrations are given here.

1. **Heart** – Hi! Heart, how are you? Hope all is well. Hey! I hope there is no obstruction in your veins. All valves working smoothly. Look I have brought plenty of oxygen for you. Enjoy! Relax!

2. **Lungs** – Hello lungs! Looking beautiful today! Feeling fresh! Yeah, I am sorry. I smoked a few cigarettes in the past. That was tough on you. But I promise, I will take good care of you now. Do let me know if you need some more fresh air. Now we are living in an airy apartment. Good oxygen here. Enjoy!

3. **Legs** – Hey legs! Looking pretty today! I know I have put on some weight. You are carrying lots of burden. I have earned my promotion too. Now there is more of travel. But I will reduce my weight. I hope your friends my knees are all fine? Enjoy! Relax!

Steps:

1. Perform Steps Number 1 to 6 as in Package Number 1 above. If time permits, you may also perform clapping and face massage for better results.

2. Now perform slow meditative 'Kapalabhati' for at least two minutes, 120 counts of exhalations.

3. This point onwards, shift your focus to left brain, continue performing 'Kapalabhati,' keeping a thought in your mind that you are exhaling to clean, cleanse and rinse your left brain, supplying oxygen only to your left brain. Mentally utter, without making any sound a few positive, assuasive, flattery-type sentences or one full pre-rehearsed paragraph for your left brain. Count ten to twenty exhalations. Remember the key points. Attention focussed on left hemisphere of brain. 'Kapalabhati' should also be involving all organs, (Hips squeezed, mild upward push/inwards squeeze on reproductive organ, belly movements, eyelid movements, etc.).

4. Repeat Step 3 for right hemisphere of brain. Count ten to twenty.

5. Repeat Step 3 for full brain, the complete mind. Count ten to twenty.

6. Repeat above for forehead, count the same. Do not forget talking to organ.

7. Repeat above for eyes. While on eyes, the force of the upward and downward squeezing, be a bit more vigorous. Eyes should feel lavation. Mind focussed on eyes. Thank them and praise them.

8. Coming to ears, catch hold of your earlobes, gently holding them between the thumb and first finger, right earlobe by right hand, and left by left hand. With each exhalation pull your earlobe down. Synchronise exhaling and pulling earlobe down. Count five to ten. (See 21.12).

9. Now catch your ears in the middle, right ear with right hand, left with left, keep arms parallel to the ground, pull ears outward. Synchronised pull with exhalations. Keep talking to ears. Count five to ten.

10. Repeat Step 9 pulling ears upwards, gripping tops of ears, right with right hand and so on.

11. While on ears you may also cross your arms, catch hold of your left earlobe with right hand and right earlobe with left hand. Pull downwards. Count five to ten. (See 21.13).

12. Repeat the same steps, involving all your important internal organs, heart, lungs, kidney, pancreas, glands, etc.

13. Now travel upwards from toe to head in the same manner, keeping important body parts in mind. Toe, legs, knee, thighs, hips, hip junctions, leg junctions, belly, torso, neck, jaws, face, forehead, etc.

14. If you are suffering from some ailment or pain in some organ, spend more time with that organ. Talk a bit longer.

15. Complete one round from head to toe for internal organs and one round from bottom to top for external organs.

16. Relax! Relax! And Relax!

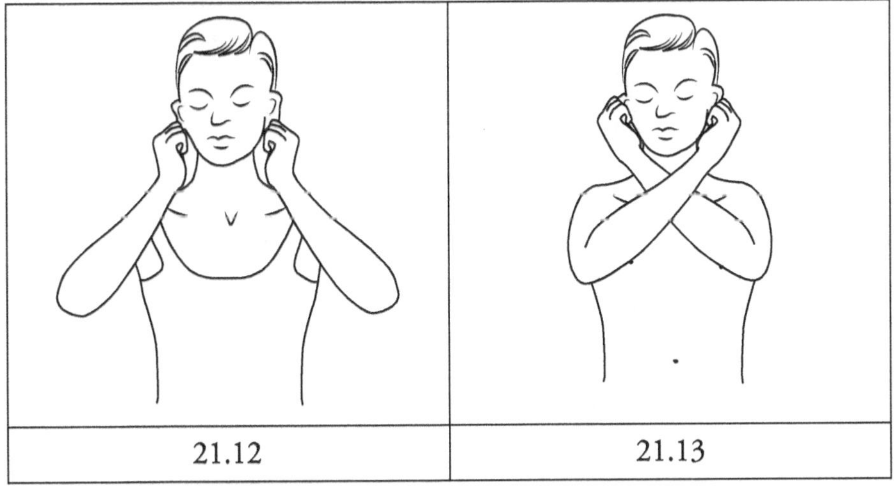

| 21.12 | 21.13 |

Day Twenty-Two: Packaged Stress Busters: Part – II

Learning and Practice for the Day

Package Number 3

This package involves tapping or massaging the body parts and some of the key points in the body. For tapping, depending upon the organ, either two fingers, i.e., index and middle fingers, or all fingers, joined together in the circular manner of right hand may be used (See 22.01). You may use tips of all fingers in both hands to tap a general area (Such as the top of skull). Do take care that your nails are properly clipped. You may also gently massage the area around the key points.

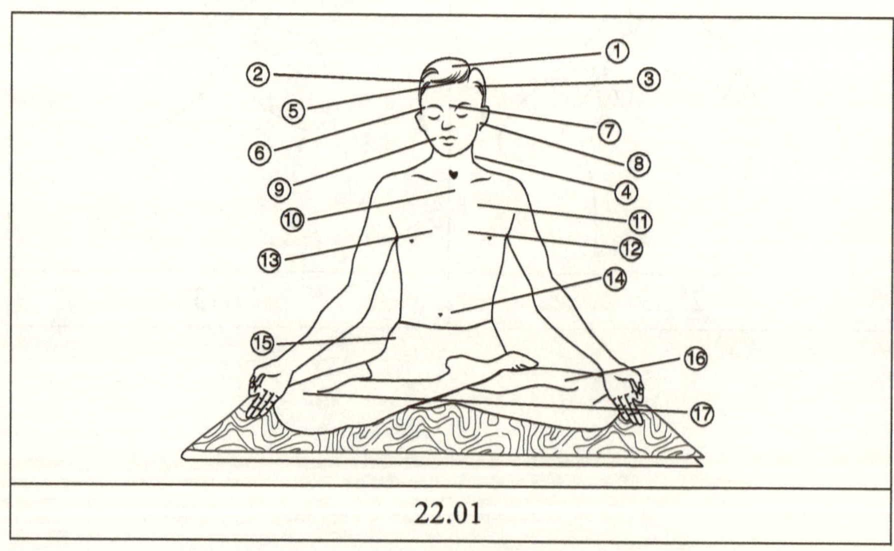

22.01

The key points to be tapped/massaged are depicted in the figure 22.01. These are:

1. Top of head, the central parting line of two hemispheres of skull.

2. Top of head, slightly protruding point in left hemisphere of skull.

3. Top of head, slightly protruding point in right hemisphere of skull.

4. Backside of neck portion, the skin surface below head and above shoulders.

5. Front of head on top line of forehead and adjoining surfaces, over forehead.

6. Two points having slight depression located between eyes and ears on left and right sides.

7. Focal point of all senses.

8. Earlobes, pointing on all three sides, i.e., downwards, upwards and sideways.

9. Face skin around dentures.

10. A point in neck where two collar bones meets.

11. A point in chest area where two ribcages separate.

12. Over the heart area.

13. Over the lungs area.

14. Navel point.

15. Hip and leg joints, both in front and back.

16. Thigh area, knees, foot joints, toes and leg fingers.

17. Tips of fingers and protruding mass at bottom of vertically aligned palms, in both hands.

Simultaneous to tapping/massaging you need to chant a mantra. Chant loudly and not merely keep it in mind. The mantra is a positive thought. You may create your own mantra. Or else you may chant,

"My body is healthy! My heart is happy!
My mind is pure! My soul is at rest!"

Synchronise the tapping with chanting of mantra, i.e., one tap for one chant.

Steps:

1. Perform Step Number 1 to 6 (or up to Step Number 17, if time permits) of Package Number 1

2. Now take both your hands upwards, forming Namaskar Mudra, give your complete body a mild upward thrust, make spine straight and head high.

<table>
<tr>
<td>

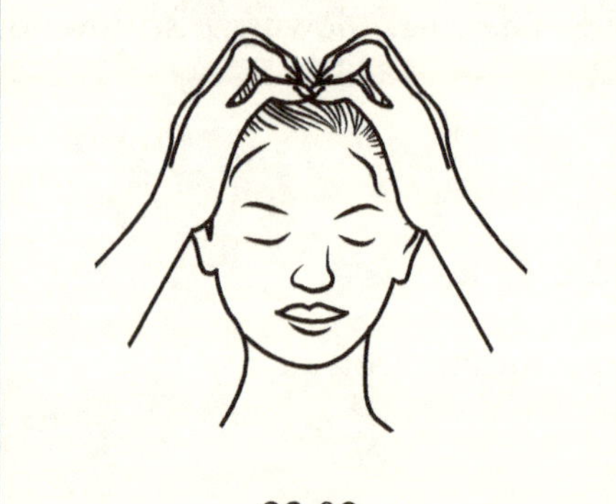

22.02

</td>
<td>

3. Now bring your hands on your head. Utilising all eight fingers of both hands, tips pointing downwards, tap on the parting line of brain hemisphere. Count twenty tappings. Keep on chanting the mantra. Breathe normally. (See 22.02).

</td>
</tr>
<tr>
<td>

4. Repeat Step 4, tapping on centre line of left hemisphere and the most upward protruding point in left side of head top surface. Count twenty tappings. Keep on chanting the mantra. (See 22.03).

</td>
<td>

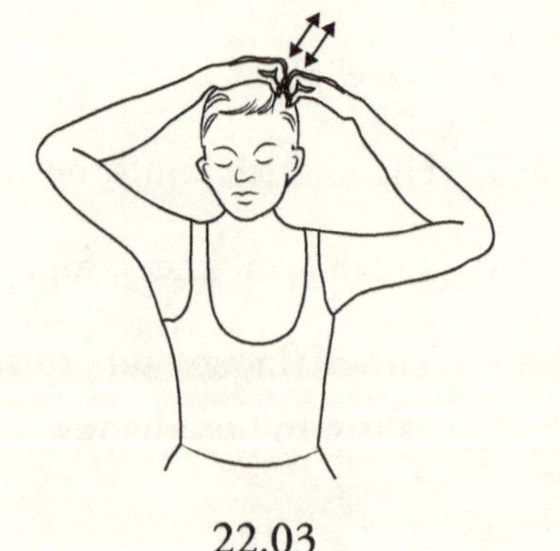

22.03

</td>
</tr>
</table>

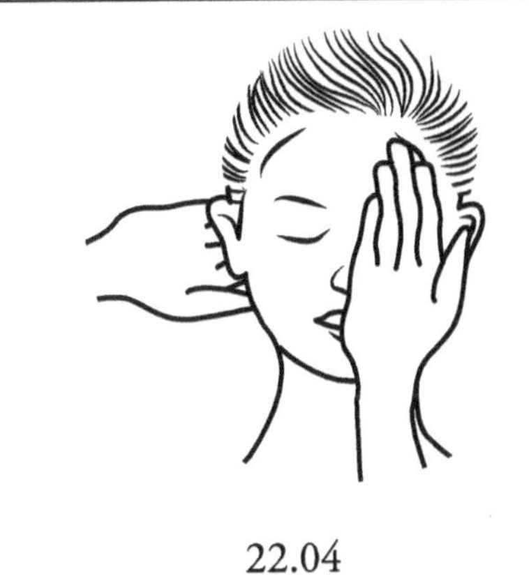

22.04

5. Place your right palm on forehead, fingers reaching the top front line of head. Place the left hand on neck. Lift the palms up. Tap on front line of head with right hand utilising all four fingers and simultaneously tap on neck portion with left hand. (See 22.04).

6. Tap with two fingers on the two points having slight depression located between eyes and ears on left and right sides. Left side with left hand and right with right hand. (See 22.05)

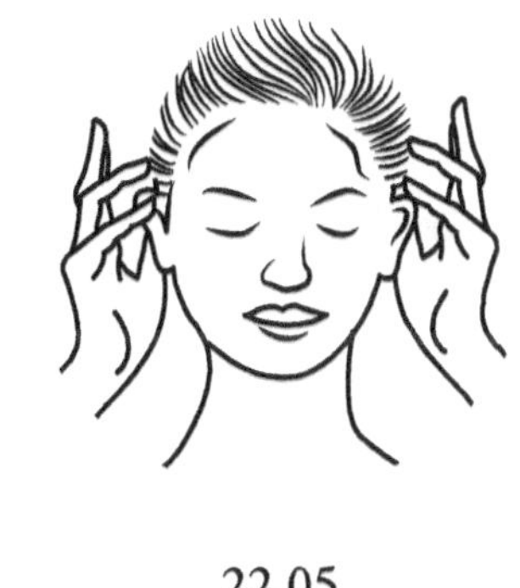

22.05

7. Similarly cover all points from head to toe. Keep on chanting the mantra.

8. Traverse your body from top to bottom and again from bottom to top in the same manner.

9. Relax.

Package Number 4: Laughter Yoga

'To laugh it off' is the best method to 'shoo away' the stress. It is now universally recognised and accepted by all healing sciences, that laughter not only cures stress and its family of bodily diseases, it also has great therapeutic effects. So, laugh your heart out! Laugh as loud as you can! Yoga has a special way for laughing. Here are the steps.

1. Stand in Tadasana. Bring a positive thought to your mind. The one that should bring a wide grin, a big smile, on your face. Loosen your complete body. Bring it to relaxed and rest stage.

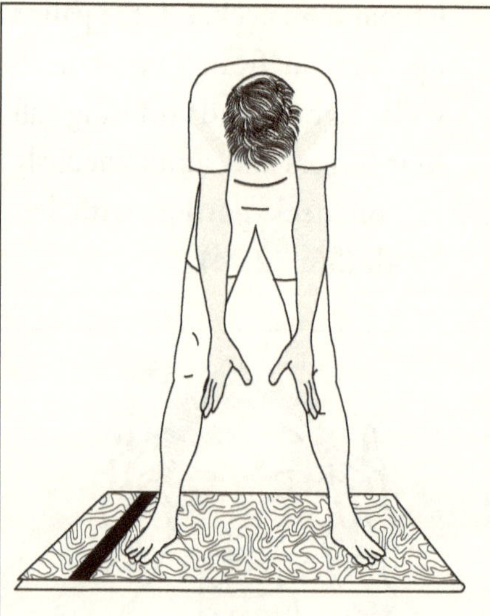

22.06

2. Now free both your hands, loosen them, tilt your body slightly in front, and take hands towards the ground as below as you can comfortably reach. (See 22.06).

3. Now laughing very, very loudly and noisily, bring your hands up, take them over your head in rotational motions, and thereafter take hands towards the back as far as you can reach. (See 22.07). Keep on laughing loud, till you run out of breath.

4. Movements of hands should be smooth, rotating on the axis of shoulders, in circular motion; try to take hands from as close to ground to as far behind your back as feasible. Your complete body should also move from bent in front, tilted in front side, to tilted in back side, along with your hands. Bring body back to central position. Stand erect. Allow breathing to be normal. Repeat Step 1 to 3 till tiredness take over and no more energy is left. Relax!

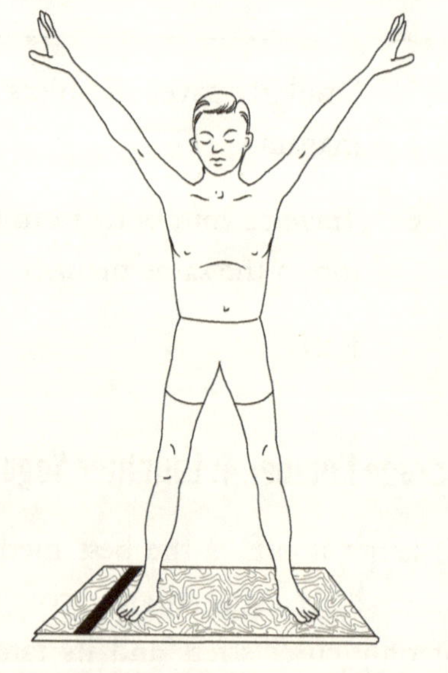

22.07

5. You may perform this laughter therapy or laughter Yoga as many times as it suits your fancy or convenience. You need not even bother about the prerequisites. No need of having a clean belly, empty bowels, timing, etc.

Other Stress Busters

1. You may also try out the combination of clapping and laughter. Sitting comfortably in any of the postures or standing loosely as in Tadasana, start laughing and clapping simultaneously. Try to bring in some elements of synchronisations between laughter and claps. After palms become red due to extra rush of bloods, perform palming of eyes and face massage. You may repeat this as many times as your hands can tolerate the mild pains of clapping. There are no prerequisites; do it whenever and wherever you get the opportunity.

2. The similar combinations of laughter, music and dancing may also be experimented with.

Day Twenty-Three: Create Your Own Package of Meditation and Pranayama

Your Own Patented Stress Buster

Now you have completed more than half of your journey on this beautiful voyage of higher learning. You have also assimilated the basics and important techniques of Meditation and Pranayama. You are fully geared up to plan and prepare a package of exercises for yourself, to be practised daily.

It is very important at this stage that from tomorrow onwards, you create a schedule. Kindly do not allow anyone else to prescribe a schedule or a package for you, howsoever learned he may be. No one understands your needs, constraints, and level of commitments to yourself better than you. You may at best seek some inspiration and some guidance at this juncture. I am only giving some guidelines here to prod you and to make your task a bit easier.

Assess Your Needs

Remember that Meditation and Pranayama are primarily focussed on relieving stresses on mind and heart (emotions). Their benefits on the physiology are incidental and bonus. You must first assess your stress levels, to create a package to relieve these stresses.

Please do not fool yourself by pretending that you do not have any stress. You cannot cure yourself if you do not confess disease. You need not assign a numerical number to your stress levels. You only must make a realistic assessment of the havoc that it is playing on your physical wellbeing, your happiness, your emotional quotient and your lifestyle.

Assess the Available Time

Once you determine the gravity of your stresses, evaluate how much time you may spare on each day, howsoever miniscule the time may be. Create a package for that much time and start practising daily. Once you get into the groove, you will yourself find, that all the constraints of time, seemingly insurmountable at the beginning, will start melting.

Stress is like cancer. Allow it to remain even in a miniscule form and slowly it will engulf the complete body. Start treating it at preliminary stage and you can easily attain victory over it. So, at first start with whatsoever time you can conveniently spare, create a package of daily, weekly and weekend day's practices. Make a strict regime. Come what may, you and your package must remain united.

Your package ideally should contain, some exercises of "Must Have" nature, some of "Should have" nature and a few of "May have" nature from the following table. If you decide on one schedule for all days, you may soon start feeling bored, repeating the same exercises every day. It is advisable to make a weekly schedule, varying the practices from "Should have" and "May have" list. Also, a bit longish and liberal package may be created for weekends. A few Yoga teachers and books prescribe a weekly rest day. If you are doing some strenuous practices, (even in Pranayama, those of intense variety), you must have one rest day in a week! For packages involving only mild and moderate practices, for ten to fifteen minutes daily, there is no need for rest day in a week.

Here are my prescriptions for "Must Have," "Should have" and "May have," just for your guidance.

Table of the Day

Serial	Practice	Minimum Time Span	Remarks
MUST HAVE (In the Beginning)			
1.	'AUM' or 'OHM' Chanting	Two Minutes, (one deep breath, three chants)	Daily
2.	Saying some prayers	One-Three Minutes	Daily
3.	Mantra Chanting	Two-Three Minutes	Daily
4.	Clapping	Two Minutes	Daily
	Meditation	One-Two Minutes	Daily
5.	Kapalabhati Pranayama	Two-Three Minutes	Daily, Slow, meditative and moderate
6.	Anuloma-Viloma Pranayama	Two-Three Minutes	Daily
(BEFORE ENDING)			
	Prayers/Mantra (Universal Peace type)	One – Two Minutes	Daily
7.	'AUM' or 'OHM' Chanting	Two Minutes, (one deep breath, three chants)	Daily
8.	Laughter Yoga	One-Two Minutes	Daily
SHOULD HAVE			
9.	Bhastrika Pranayama	Two-Three Minutes	Minimum three days in a week
10.	Bhramari Pranayama	Two-Three Minutes	Minimum two days in a week
11.	One or Two of Advanced Pranayama technique	Two-Three Minutes	Include one for each day of a week

MAY HAVE			
12.	Fun breathing exercises	Four-Five Minutes	For weekend days initially
13.	Packaged stress busters	As per time of package	For weekend days
14.	Prolonged laughter session	Five-Ten Minutes	For weekend days

Congratulations, for discovering the cure for the emotional cancer of your body!

Congratulations, for discovering the cure for the stress in your life!

Chapter-Four

The Subtle Exercises
(Yogic Sukshma-Vyayama)

Day Twenty-Four: Yogic Sukshma–Vyayama (The Subtle Exercises)

Learning for the Day

Introduction

'Sukshma-Vyayama,' a 'Sanskrit' word, literally translates into 'The subtle exercises.' These are easier exercises and may be practised by anyone, advanced or beginner, elderly or young and also by those recuperating from or suffering from some moderate ailments.

This series of exercises is also referred to as 'Pawanmukta' series. 'Pawan' means 'Wind' or 'Prana'; 'Mukta' means 'Release' and 'Asana,' as is obvious, means 'Pose' or 'Posture.' Therefore 'Pawanmukta' series of 'asana' means those groups of Asanas that remove any blockages which prevent the free flow of air, fluids and energy in the body and the mind.

In our normal day-to-day working, due to adoption of bad postures, disturbances in body functioning, inverted and imbalanced lifestyles and psychological and emotional problems, the flows of winds, fluids or energy gets blocked.

This initially results into stiffening, muscular tensions, improper blood flows, and subtle functional defects. However, sustained, chronic and persistent blockages may result into a limb, joint or physical organ malfunctioning or acquiring some disease.

Regular practising of this series of Asana removes such existing blockages from the body and prevents new formations of blockages. This way, the series promotes total health, regulating, streamlining and stabilizing the flows throughout the body.

Human body also contains many joints, pinions, ratchets and bearings requiring regular lubrication. This lubrication process is also automatic and self-sustaining. Some organs bear the burden of lubricating the other organs. This series promotes smoothening and enhancing such lubricating actions also.

This series is one of the most important series of practices, having profound effects on body and mind. Thus, it is an important tool for Yogic management (prevention, cleanings, periodic maintenance and lubrications) of various disorders, and maintenance of health.

The credit for development, achieving perfection, promotions and promulgation of this part of Yoga, rightfully goes to 'Bihar School of Yoga.' The 'Sukshma-Vyayama' series also have many variations and sub-categorisations. Instead of giving too much of theory, I would like to lead you to start your practices by understanding some more basics. These are:

- These Asanas relax the muscles of the body. The relaxing impulses travel back to the brain and relax the mind. Therefore, involvement of both mind and body, in a synchronised and harmonious manner is very important. By integrating the breath synchronisation and focus of mind and senses, the attentive faculty of mind is made active. Mind is not allowed to wander into stresses and tensions.

- The overall effect is thus more mental, than physical. These Asanas relax the mind, tune up the autonomic nerves, hormonal functions and tone up other actions and activities of internal organs.

- Some group of Asanas work on physical structures of bones, joints, etc. (named as Anti-Rheumatic Groups). Some works on digestion and abdomen (Digestive/abdominal group) and some on energy blockages (The Energy Block Group). All supplement and complement each other.

- They stimulate and encourage free flow of energies throughout the body. It is therefore important to understand the intricacies and minute points of each practice and perfect the posture to derive maximum benefit. Before attempting advanced YogaAsanas, which are often physically demanding, the practitioner is advised to perfect the postures of this series. Sustained practice will bring profound relaxation and toning up of entire psycho-physiological structure and prepare the practitioner for advanced Asanas.

- These exercises may be performed with focus of mind and senses in three ways: first— with focus on actual physical activity, second— with focus of senses and integrated breathing, and third—with focus of movements of 'prana' in the body. Only after you start practising and do some hits and trials, will you come to know the subtle differences and intricacies of each.

- These exercises are recommended to be performed in sequential manner, i.e., one after the other as prescribed and described, covering all major parts of the body and the joints systems.

- Most text books recommend starting from toes and going up to the head. Since these are joint freeing exercises, start with freeing the joints of bottom parts of body (toes) and finish after freeing the joints in upper parts of the body (neck).

- However, based on my own personal experiences, I recommend that loosening joints in lower parts of spinal systems, particularly the joints in lower back should take precedence. I am covering these loosening (joint freeing exercises for spine) up front. You may later conduct your own hits and trials and may include the spinal series in middle or end.

- Do not start practising these exercises straightaway after leaving the bed. These are Yogic routines and all prerequisites are required to be strictly followed.

- On their face they may look simple, sweet and innocent but are very powerful. Prepare and prime your body before starting. If you are short on time and cannot plan a proper Meditation-Pranayama schedule, start with at least simple inhalation-exhalations Pranayama. Inhale through the nostrils, slowly and steadily, without making any sound, then exhale slowly, continuously and silently. Have inhalations and exhalations for same durations (may be ten seconds each). Do this for at least twenty-five times. This will improve concentration and enable you to synchronise breathing with actions.

- For some exercises ten to twelve repetitions/rounds are prescribed. This prescription is applicable for a healthy male, in the prime of his youth. Depending upon your age and health conditions, the number of repetitions may be reduced. However, maintain minimum count of three. Also keep in mind the basics of periodic rest, relax after completing one round in relaxation posture and shift to relaxation posture/Shavasana at the slightest hint of tiredness and pain.

Practice for the Day

Continue your own package of practices for Meditation and Pranayama. By now you are expected to master all the practices of your own package.

Day Twenty-Five: The Subtle Exercises for Spinal System: Part – I

Learning and Practices for the Day

Everyone, even those having only rudimentary knowledge of human physiology, should be aware that the spine and associated systems of bone structure, muscles and nerves are the most complex and most important body systems.

This is the system responsible for distinguishing humans from other animals. We are able to stand on our feet and walk with head held high. This system is also most vulnerable to ill effects of distorted lifestyles and effects of ageing. Majority of lifestyle diseases and age-related ailments can be taken care of by taking appropriate care of this system.

That is primarily the reason for keeping this section ahead of all other 'Sukshma-Vyayama.' Let us understand and start practising for taking some very good care of our spinal system.

We will begin with reiterating the starting posture (base position or 'Prarambhiksthiti'). Recollect Posture Number S1 from Day-Nine Chapter-One's learnings. It is advisable that you warm up your body a little bit by performing your own Meditation and Pranayama routine exercises, before starting these subtle exercises. Also remember synchronising your breathings with exercise and focus of mind.

The Starting Posture: (Base Position)

Sit with the legs outstretched. Place the palms of the hands on the floor to the sides and just behind the buttocks. The back, neck and head should be straight. Straighten the elbows. Lean back slightly, taking the support of the arms. Close the eyes and relax the whole body in this position. This is also referred to as 'PRARAMBHIKSTHITI.'

Exercise Number 25.01: LOOSENING THE JOINTS IN LOWER BACK

Steps:

1. Sit in starting posture, the base posture, i.e., Prarambhiksthiti, or the base position.

2. Release your hands and push the upper part of the body towards the front, making the spine vertical to the surface, and join both legs. Breathe normally.

<table>
<tr>
<td>

3. Now fold your right leg inwards, with the help and support of both hands. Bring your right leg, such that the right heel is placed at the parting line of hips in front, just beneath the reproductive organ. Breathe normally. (See 25.01)

</td>
<td>

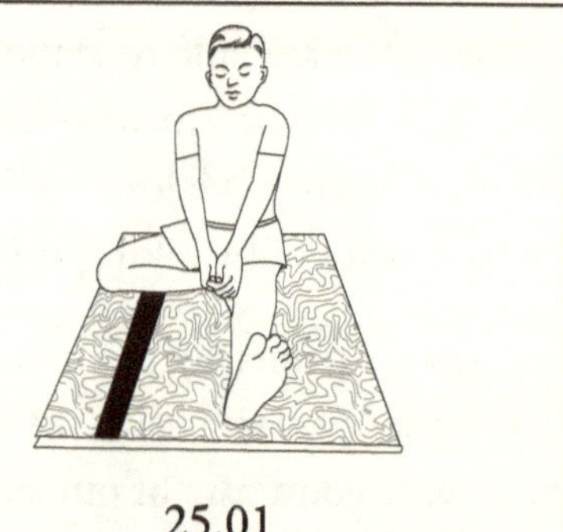

25.01

</td>
</tr>
<tr>
<td>

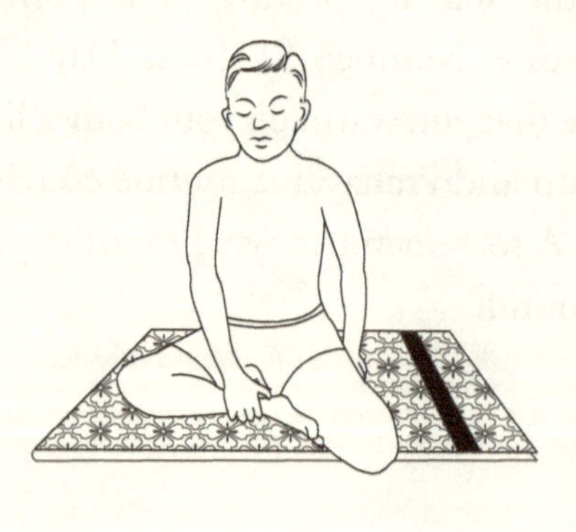

25.02

</td>
<td>

4. Now taking support of hands, fold your left leg outwards, and bring it behind your buttocks, toes pointed and facing away from body, heel touching the parting line of hips in backside. Relax, breathe normally. Try to align both feet in same line, right in front and left in backside. (See 25.02)

</td>
</tr>
</table>

5. Now take both your hands upwards, hands folded in Namaskar Mudra, and take them over your head, stretching mildly upwards. Relax and give one mild upward stretch coupled with one deep inhalation. (See 25.03)

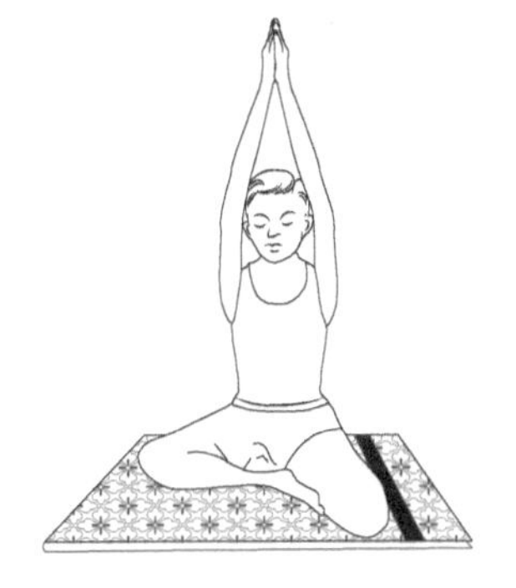

25.03

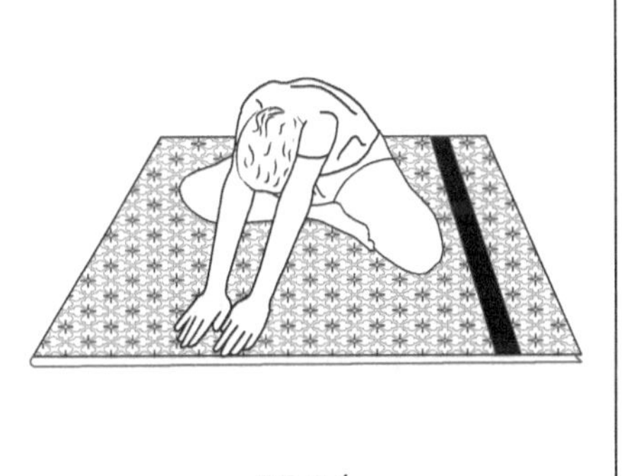

25.04

6. Sitting in this position, exhale and start moving your complete upper body towards front side, so that your palms touch the floor surface, fingers pointing outwards, try to touch your nose with the surface. If difficult, bring it as close to the surface as feasible. (See 25.04)

7. Your abdominal area, chest, face all in same line, should as far as possible, be touching the surface. Stretch your hands in front, as far away from the buttocks as feasible. Feel mild stretch in the lower spine and at spine-hip joint. Breathe normally and stay in this posture for ten to twenty seconds (twenty counts of breathings). Focus attention on spine-hip joint.

8. Release this posture by slowly taking your hands, head, chest and abdomen upwards. Form Namaskar Mudra with hands. After releasing the posture and making hands free, bring left leg from back side to front side and take it in front as it was in base position. Take your right leg also in base position. Relax and breathe normally in base position.

9. Now repeat the same steps the other way, i.e., by folding the left leg inwards, placing left heel below hips in front, and folding the right leg outwards, taking right heel below buttocks in back. Then taking complete body in front, resting in posture for ten to twenty seconds and thereafter releasing the posture.

10. This completes one routine. You may initially practise by performing three to four routines.

11. Persons used to long hours of working, while sitting on chairs, are likely to develop stiffness in spine-hips joint. Sustained stiffness results in lower back pains. This exercise removes this stiffness. One routine of this exercise must be included in your daily practice.

Exercise Number 25.02: ROTATIONAL MOVEMENTS OF HANDS AND HEAD

In this exercise we will rotate both our arms, sideways, causing pendulum like circular movements. We will also rotate our head and neck sideways. Head and hands will go in opposite directions.

When hands are rotating and going rightwards, neck and head will go leftwards, and vice-versa. You may form a fist, joining both your hands at palm or you may keep them apart, as found comfortable.

Steps:

1. Sitting in base position, and preferably immediately after performing Exercise Number 25.01, take both your hands, in pendulum like movements, towards the right side, shoulders forming the pivot points, force them as far as feasible in backward direction.

2. Simultaneous to this movement of hands, rotate your neck, and bring your head in leftwards direction. Try to stretch your head backwards, in an apparent effort to see your back side, up to as far as neck can conveniently take your head. (See 25.05)

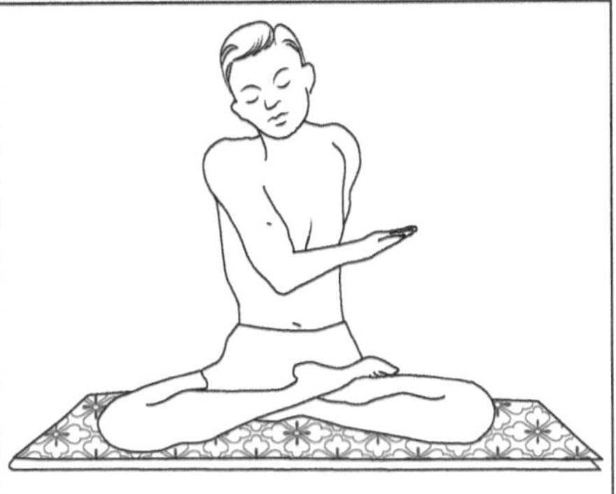

25.05

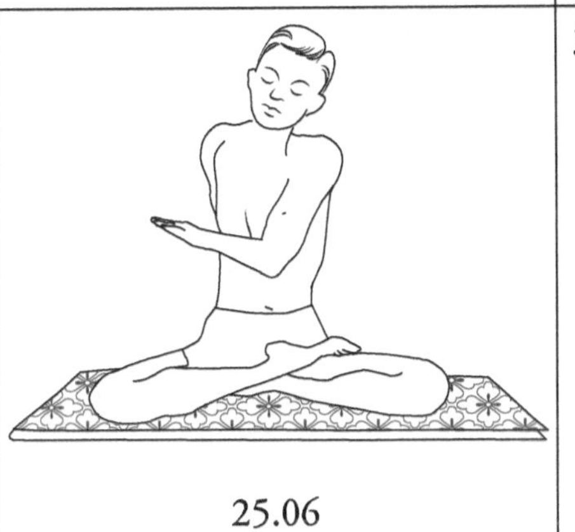

25.06

3. After your hands reach the extreme position on right side and head on left side, bring your hands from this position to the extreme position in other direction, i.e., on left side, also simultaneously take head in extreme position on right side. (See 25.06)

4. All movements of hands, the neck and head must be smooth. No jerks. Breathing should be synchronised, when head is travelling from centre position towards left, it is time to inhale. When head reaches the central position in front, time to exhale. Attention be focussed on movements of hands and neck, and rotational stresses in spine-hip joints.

5. Repeat the exercise for ten to twelve times, counting movement in one direction as one count.

Exercise Number 25.03: THE MARJARI ASANA (CAT POSTURE)

Have you ever experienced jealousy for your girlfriend's pet cat for being the centre point of her love and affection? I cannot help you in the matters of love and affection of your girlfriend. You must earn it yourself. But I can make you feel like a cat. You may make movements of your body, like a cat, and thus derive benefits for your spine. Here are the steps:

Steps:

1. Sit in any easier variant of Vajrasana (Posture Number S2, Chapter-One, Day-Nine). Breathe normally and relax in this posture.

2. Now take both your hands upwards, over your head, palms facing in front. Exhaling, shift your complete body weight smoothly in front taking support of your hands and bring your body supported on four limbs, elbows placed near the knees. Back portion supported on knees and legs, and upper body weight supported on elbows and hands. Palms facing downwards. Feel like a cat. (See 25.07).

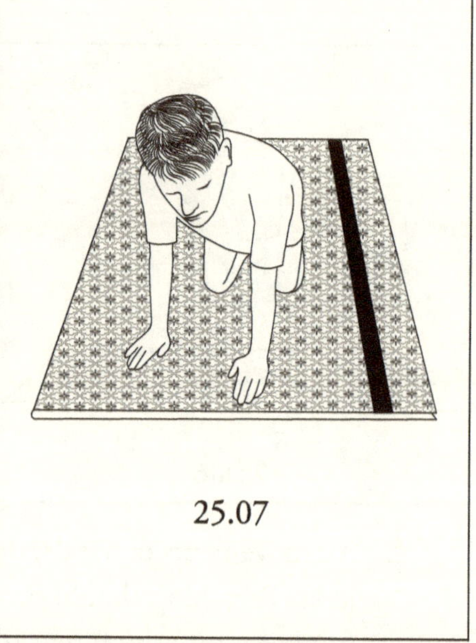

25.07

3. Now making a smooth movement, using palm and fingers, shift your palms, six inches ahead in front. Shifting your complete body weight also about six inches ahead smoothly, lift your back and smoothly balance the body weight on four limbs, two palms and two knees. Relax in this posture for three to five seconds, breathing normally.

4. Now from this posture, we will move the head and upper torso upwards in front with inhalation and downwards towards chest coupled with exhalation. When the head will go upwards the spine will be pushed downwards to form a concave shape. Similarly, when head goes downwards, spine will be consciously pushed upwards, to form a convex shape, with centre point of spine to be at top most height. (See 25.08)

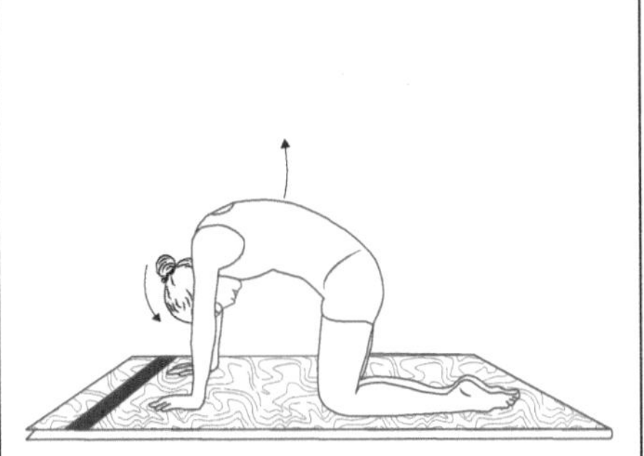

25.08

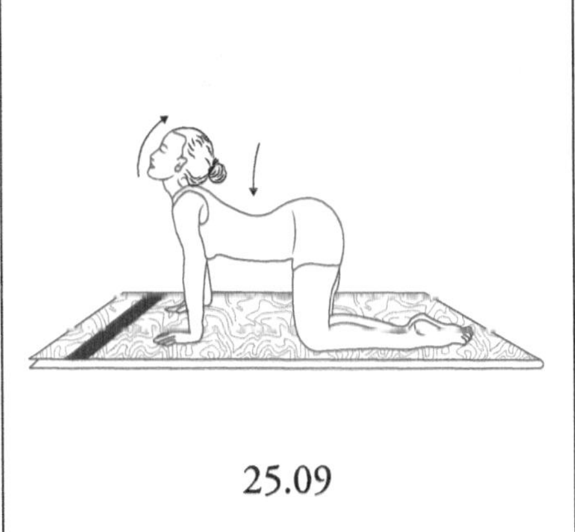

25.09

5. Let your chin touch the collarbone in your chest, when moving downwards. Let head go as high as feasible in upwards movements. All movements be smooth. No jerks. Try to form as sharp a convex and concave shape with spine, in downwards and upwards movements of head, as feasible. Head movement will also cause shifting complete body weights slightly in forwards and backwards directions. (See 25.09)

6. Try to restrict the movements of spine in forward and backward directions. Spine should only smoothly change shape from convex to concave positions, without unnecessarily moving in front and backward directions. No movements of body should also occur

towards left or right sides. During the forward movements of body and upwards movement of head inhale deeply. Exhale forcefully during the downwards movements of head. Retain the breath during holding the posture in convex and concave shapes.

7. Remember the steps carefully. Inhale; move head upwards, form concave shape with spine, try to bring centre point of spine as close to ground as feasible. All smooth. Exhale, move head downwards, form a convex shape with spine, try to take centre point of spine as up as feasible. Attention should be focussed on movements of spine and stretch being felt at spine-hip joint and neck-head joints. Repeat ten to twelve times, counting one cycle of upward and downward movement as one count.

8. You may also look at this posture from the prism of your knowledge of dancing puppets, held with strings tied to the fingers of the puppeteer. Imagine that a puppeteer is holding your back tied with a rope/string and pulling you up from the middle of spine and then letting you down. This way you may perfect the convex and concave formations of spine.

9. If still in any doubt, closely observe a dog or cat, immediately after it awakens from sleep. The first thing these animals do is to exercise their spine, by making a few concave and convex formations with spine, neck and head. These animals are not only good pets; they may be good teachers too. After all, unless adopted, they must remain healthy without any support of Vets.

Day Twenty-Six: The Subtle Exercises for Spinal System: Part – II

Learning and Practices for the Day

Exercise Number 26.01: SPINAL UPWARDS TRIANGULAR STRETCH

Steps:

1. Lie down comfortably on your back. Relax in Shavasana (Supine Posture-Base position).

2. Fold both of your legs and place heels touching the buttocks, toes pointing outwards. Tilt your head slightly inwards, towards the hips, stretching the neck slightly. The position of head should be such that you get good contact surface below your head. You need more surface to balance the weight of upper body. Your eyes should be seeing an object on ceiling/sky placed vertically up and slightly behind you.

3. Now keeping spine straight and inhaling deeply, raise your hips, forming a smooth triangle with your spine. Your body weight should be uniformly supported on three pressure points, head, toes or heels. Arms should be performing the functions of ensuring stability of the posture, i.e., not allowing body to fall abruptly towards left or right side. Stay in this posture for five to ten seconds. Return back to normal position. Breathing be synchronised with actions. Inhale when taking hips in upward direction, retain when

holding the posture, and exhale while bringing hips downwards. Attention be focussed on spinal and hip movements and spinal stretches. Repeat ten to twelve times.

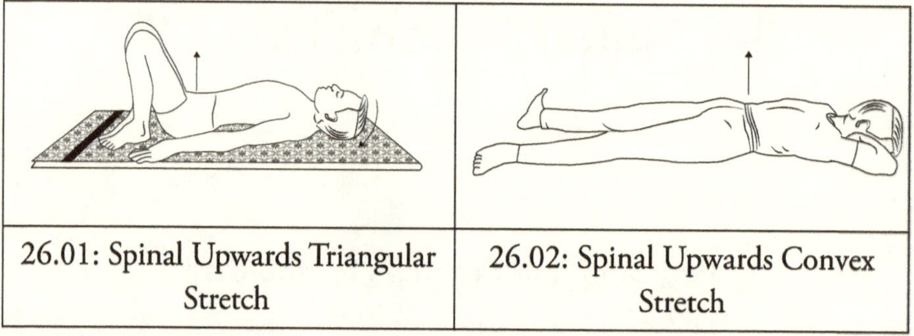

26.01: Spinal Upwards Triangular Stretch	26.02: Spinal Upwards Convex Stretch

Exercise Number 26.02: SPINAL UPWARDS CONVEX STRETCH

Steps:

1. Lie down flat on your stomach (Posture Number R2, Prone Posture). Relax in any of the relaxation postures.

2. Place your right hand palm beneath your forehead, palm facing downwards. Now place the left hand palm facing downwards over right hand palm. Making a pillow like formation with both palms, place your forehead on this palm-formation. Keep head slightly tilted inwards, i.e., neck tilted towards the chest and the ground. From this posture, inhaling deeply, consciously try to lift your hips slightly in upwards direction by a few inches.

3. Try it to the extent of reaching a posture wherein your hips are raised as high as feasible, and body weight gets uniformly balanced on your two big toes and head (placed on hands). Spine will thus form a convex shape with head and toes acting as endpoints of this convex formation and hip the central point. Initially it may be difficult to attain this posture. Start with balancing your

body weight on head and knees and gradually try to perfect the posture.

4. Breathings be synchronised. Inhale when forming the convex, retain when holding and exhale when taking spine down. Do not over try. You may cause injury to spine, if downward movement takes place by actions of gravity, or a thud-like abrupt fall takes place, due to not exercising due care and precaution. The upwards movement of hips by a few inches looks subtle and easy. However even a minor fall from stretched condition of spine may cause injury. Beware; you are dealing with very sensitive parts of your body.

5. Single pointed focus of attention must be on spine. Unless you channelize your mental energy of brain to action, it is not feasible to smoothly form a convex shape with spine. Also, mind must guide all organs properly in releasing the posture smoothly and properly.

6. Relax in any relaxation posture. You may perform ten to twelve repetitions.

Exercise Number 26.03: NECK-SPINE JOINT EXERCISE

This exercise is to be performed while lying down on your belly, face down (Prone posture). The steps are:

1. Lie down on your belly. Attain Posture Number R4, the crocodile pose (i.e., Makrasana). Relax in this posture.

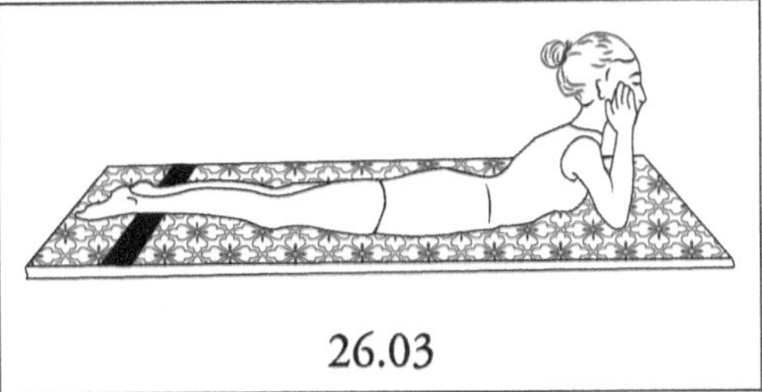

26.03

2. Now lift your head slightly upwards by about six inches to

one foot. (This posture is akin to Bhujangasana). Folds your arms upwards, such that the elbows remain touching on ground. Hands should be forming Namaskar Mudra, fingers pointing upwards. Now open your fingers, bottom of palms touching each other, and form a cuplike shape (shape of English alphabet "U"). Allow your face to be encased in hollow formed between your palms, such that your chin is resting on joints of the palms-bottoms. Head and spine must be in straight line, making an obtuse angle with leg-lines. (See 26.03)

Taking support of the hands, smoothly move the head in left and right directions. (See 26.04). Both palms and head should move together, elbows firmly resting, bottom of neck and neck-spine joint should feel mild stretch. Maintain breath synchronisation, exhaling slowly in central position and inhaling when head is moving towards left or right. Repeat ten to twelve times. Relax!

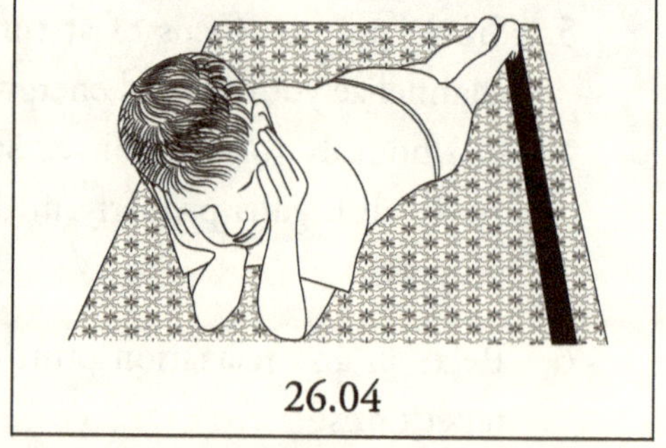

26.04

3. Now release your face from the palm-formation of hands. Retain the palm-formation to enable supporting the head, in case of mild downwards jerks, if any. Smoothly move the head in upwards and downwards directions, the neck-spine joint working like a pivot. Allow your chin to kiss the collarbone in downwards extreme position. Repeat ten to twelve times. Do not cause any abrupt movements. Inhale when head goes high and exhale when it is coming down. Relax!

4. Retaining the same posture, rotate the head, in clockwise direction, in small circular motions, to form a circle of very small diameter, with neck-spine joint acting as centre point of circular motion. Repeat ten to twelve times.

5. Repeat Step Number 5 with head moving in anti-clockwise direction. Repeat ten to twelve times.

There are many other postures, exercises and Asanas in Yoga, immensely benefitting the spinal systems. Some (very few) shall be described later in Chapter-Five.

Day Twenty-Seven: The Subtle Exercises for Legs: Part – I

Learning and Practice for the Day

The organs that distinguish animal life from plant life are legs and feet. Animals are mobile, plants are not. Mobility is an important bliss for humans too. Even small hindrances in mobility are troublesome. It transforms human life into plant life. Age also plays its first havoc on legs.

The pain in knee joints is the most common age-related ailment. We may prolong the useful life of our legs, by just devoting ten to fifteen minutes every day, routinely and dedicatedly. Even if you are not a Yoga enthusiast, your fitness regime must include exercising your legs. This will ensure that the quality of life even in the sunset phase of your life remains satisfactory, if not great. Yoga, of course, contains a package of practices to ensure good quality of life, even at the age of eighty plus. So, let us start the Yogic way of looking after our legs.

Remember the key points of starting posture (base position), synchronise breathings with movements, focus of attention and performing all exercises in this series in sequential manner.

Exercise Number 27.01: THE TOE BENDING EXERCISE

In this exercise, to-and-fro movements of big toes and other toes are caused.

Steps:

1. Sit in the base position with the legs outstretched and the feet slightly apart. Place the hands beside and slightly behind the buttocks.

2. Lean back a little, using the arms to support the back. Keep the spine as straight as possible. Focus attention on the toes. Keep toes pointed. Move the toes of both feet slowly backwards and forwards, keeping the feet upright and the ankles relaxed and motionless.

3. The smaller toes should also accompany the big toe in all movements. When big toe is moving in front direction, try and join all other toes together. When big toe is moving in backwards directions the other toes should be separated and well spread out.

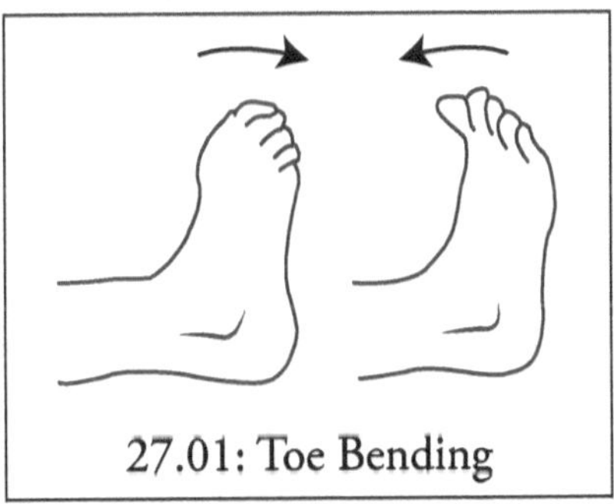

27.01: Toe Bending

4. Hold each position for a few seconds. Repeat ten to twelve times. This exercise is also called as 'PADANGULI NAMAN'and 'GOOLF NAMAN.'

5. **Breathing:** Inhale as the toes move backwards. Exhale as the toes move forward.

6. **Focus: Mind:** On the breath, mentally counting the breathings and movements and focussed on the stretching sensation produced by the movement. Eyes: Preferably closed or focussed on the toes, tracing and guiding the toes movements.

7. After some practise, you should notice that this innocent looking minor exercise of just bending the toes, stretches your muscles and nerves from neck down to the hips along the backbone and from hips to toes and foot-fingers. That is the power of Yoga. Appreciate it.

Exercise Number 27.02: THE ANKLE BENDING EXERCISE

In this to-and-fro movement of feet, with ankle acting as hinge, no external support shall be caused.

Steps:

1. Remain in the base position. Keep the feet slightly apart.

2. Slowly move both feet backward and forward, bending them from the ankle joints. Try to stretch the feet forward to enable the big toes to touch the floor and then draw them back towards the knees. Knees should remain still, fixed in place and as stationary as feasible.

3. If it is difficult to keep the knees stationary initially, you may place your palms on knees, to keep them in position and thus perfect the posture with gradual practice.

4. Hold each position for a few seconds. Repeat ten to twelve times. This is known as 'GOOLF NAMAN.'

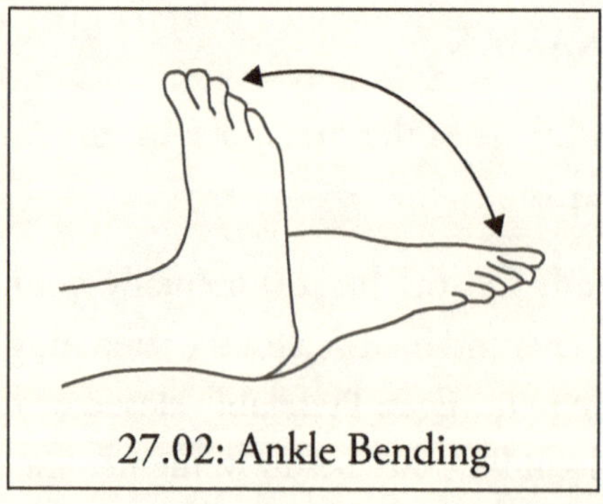

27.02: Ankle Bending

5. **Breathing:** Inhale as the foot moves forward to make attempt to touch the floor with big toe. Exhale as the foot moves backwards.

6. **Focus: Mind:** On the breath, mentally counting the breathings and the movements, also focussed on the stretch in the foot, ankle, calf and leg muscles or joints. Eyes: Preferably closed or focussed on the ankles, closely observing and guiding the movements.

Exercise Number 27.03: THE ANKLE ROTATION EXERCISE

1. Remain in the base position. Separate the legs a little, keeping them straight. Keep the heels on the ground throughout the practice.

2. **Rotation Number 1:** Slowly rotate the right foot clockwise from the ankle ten to twelve times and then repeat ten to twelve times anti-clockwise. Repeat the same procedure with the left foot. (See 27.03)

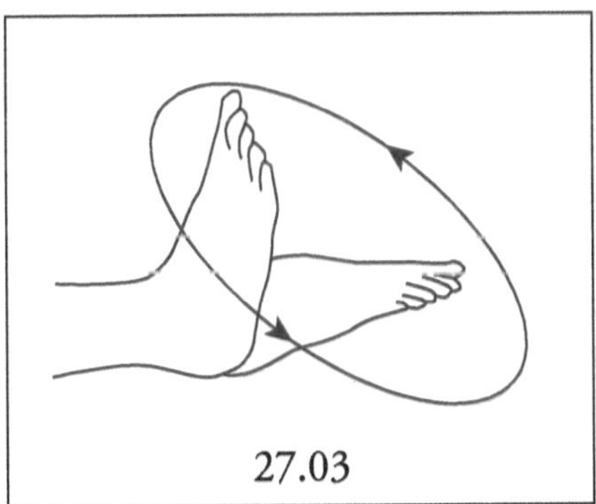

27.03

3. **Rotation Number 2:** Place the feet together. Slowly rotate both feet together in the same direction, keeping them in contact with each other. Do not allow the knees to move. Practise ten to twelve times clockwise and then ten to twelve times anti-clockwise. (See 27.04)

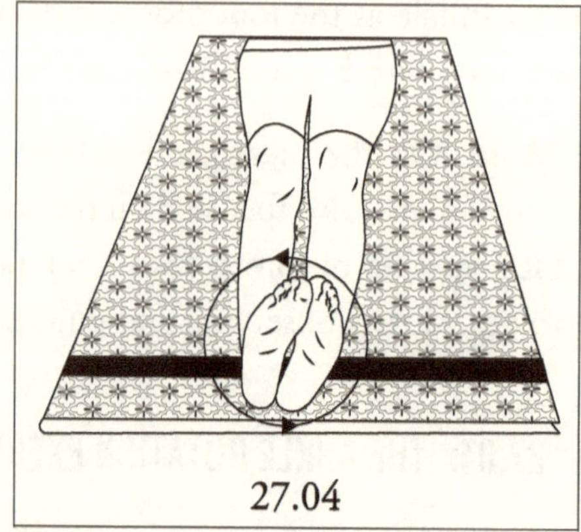

27.04

4. **Rotation Number 3:** Keep the feet separated by about one foot. Slowly rotate both feet from the ankles together but in opposite directions. The big toes should touch each other on the inward stroke of each foot. Do ten to twelve rotations in one direction and then ten to twelve rotations in the opposite direction. (See 27.05)

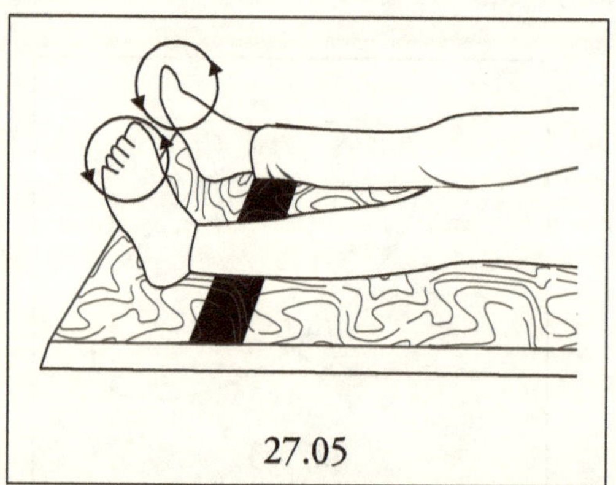

27.05

5. This exercise is also referred to as 'GOOLF CHAKRA.'

6. **Breathing:** Inhale on the upward movement. Exhale on the downward movement.

7. **Focus: Mind:** Focussed on the breath, mentally counting the rotations and the breathings. Eyes may be closed or focussed on the toes observing and guiding movements.

Exercise Number 27.04: THE KNEECAP CONTRACTION EXERCISE

Steps:

1. Stay in the basic sitting posture. Contract the muscle surrounding the right knee, drawing the kneecap back towards the thigh. (See 27.06). Hold the contraction for three to five seconds, counting mentally.

2. Release the contraction and let the kneecap return to its normal position. Practise five times. Repeat with the left kneecap five times, then with both kneecaps together. The name of this exercise as per 'Bihar School of Yoga' is 'JANUFALAK AKARSHAN.'

3. **Breathing:** Inhale while contracting. Hold the breath during contraction. Exhale while relaxing the knee muscles.

4. **Focus:** Mind: On the breath, mentally counting each contraction and release. Eyes: Preferably closed or focussed on the knee/knees, keenly observing the contraction and release of compression on knee/knees.

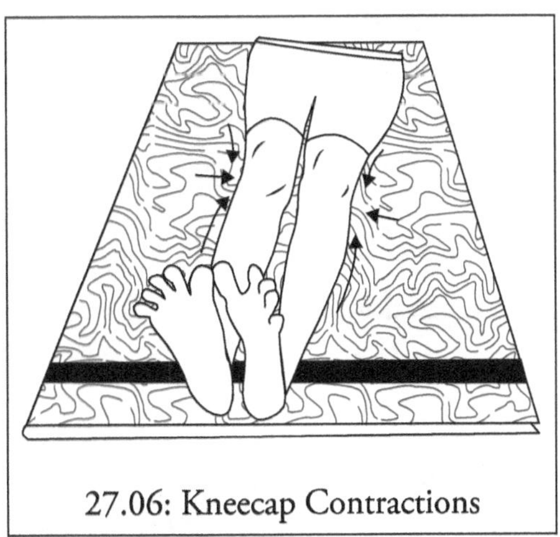

27.06: Kneecap Contractions

Day Twenty-Eight: The Subtle Exercises for Legs: Part – II

Learning and Practice for the Day

Continuing our learning from the previous day, we will learn and practise a few more of the subtle exercises, i.e., the 'Sukshma-Vyayama' beneficial for our legs. Today's exercises are to be performed in sequential manner after completing the exercises learnt yesterday.

Exercise Number 28.01: THE HANDS WARMINGUP EXERCISE: CHOPPING UP SOME WOOD

Next few routines require use of hands. It is therefore necessary that we warm them up and make them ready to be involved in the exercises. So! How about warming up with chopping some wood! This exercise involves moving the hands forcefully up and down, as if using an axe (Hindi: Kulhadhi-Sanchalan) for wood chopping.

Steps:

1. Sitting in base position, free your hands, make spine straight and vertical.

2. Form a close fist, with both hands joined together, fingers of hands interlocked, inserting each finger of the right hand, in the space between the two adjacent fingers of the left hand, closely and forcefully closing the fist. Imagine that you are holding an axe between your palms.

3. Now take both your hands forcefully up, in a circular motion, as high as you can. Hold. (See 28.01). Now bring them down with full force, imagining a wooden plank, ready to be chopped, placed on the chopping block in front of you. Chop the wood with full force. (See 28.02)

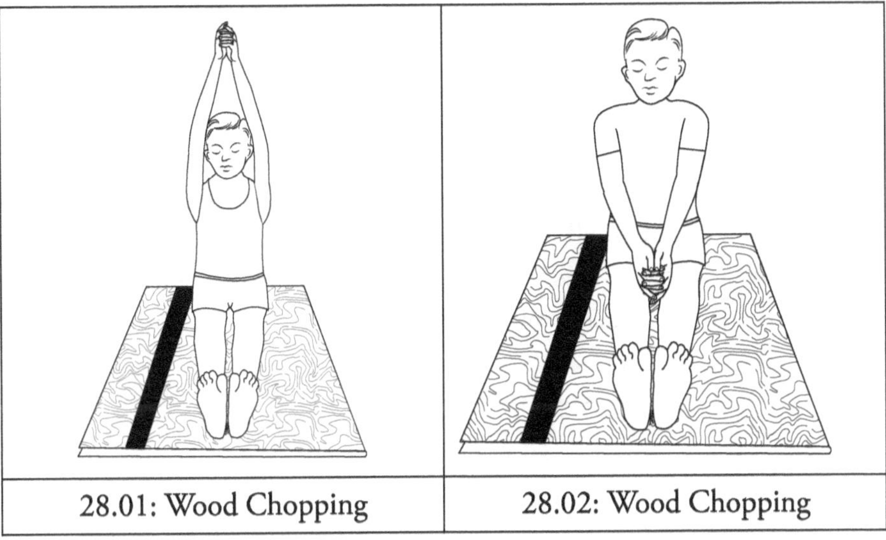

| 28.01: Wood Chopping | 28.02: Wood Chopping |

4. Repeat the up and down movements for ten to twelve times. Relax till the breathing is normal.

5. **Breathing:** Inhale on the upward movement. Exhale forcefully on the downward movement.

6. **Focus: Mind:** On the breath, mentally counting the up and down movements. Eyes: May be closed or focussed on the hands at the fist point.

Exercise Number 28.02: THE KNEE MOVEMENTS EXERCISE

In this we will exercise the leg-hip joint and the knee joint, by causing to-and-fro movements of leg. Both joints working as hinges should get lubricated. This exercise is also referred to as 'JANU NAMAN' or 'GHOOTNA CHALANA.'

Steps:

1. Immediately after completing the Exercise Number 28.01 above and following the mandatory relaxation phase, start this exercise.

2. Bend your right leg, slightly upwards, lifting knee up, right foot remaining on ground. Insert your right hand beneath right thigh from right hand side. Now, also insert your left hand below right thigh from left hand side and catch complete hold of thigh by interlocking fingers of both hands, thus forming the grip.

3. With the firm support of hand grip, push the thigh and right leg upwards, in an effort, so that the right knee reaches the tip of the nose, without bending the neck forward. Even if you are not able to make contact between the knee and the nose, bring them as close as feasible.

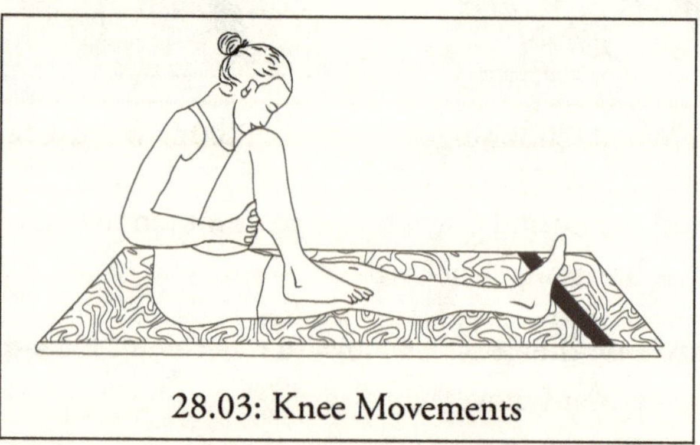

28.03: Knee Movements

4. The belly should experience good amount of compression on right side. The knee joint should experience about 120-degree rotational movement on its axis. The thigh-hip joint experiences approximately 90-degree rotational movement on its axis.

5. Hold this posture for five to ten seconds. Release and allow leg to straighten up, moving in front. Retain the hand grip beneath the thigh.

6. Repeat this to-and-fro movement of leg ten to twelve times.

7. Repeat the same steps for left leg for ten to twelve rounds, relaxing in between as required.

8. **Breathing:** Inhale on the forward movement of leg. Exhale on the backward movement. Retain when holding the knee close to nose.

9. **Focus: Mind:** On the breath, mentally counting to-and-fro movements or breathings. Eyes may be closed or focussed on the knee.

Exercise Number 28.03: THE DOUBLE KNEE BENDING EXERCISE

Precautions:

This is a strenuous practice and should not be attempted by people with weak abdominal muscles, back conditions, high blood pressure or heart conditions.

Steps:

1. Sitting in the base position, place both palms flat on the floor at the sides and slightly in front of the buttocks. Bend both knees together and place the feet on the floor in front of the buttocks.

2. Straighten the legs and raise the feet so that they are about 8 cm above the floor in the final position. Point the toes forward. The hands and arms should support and maintain stability of the body.

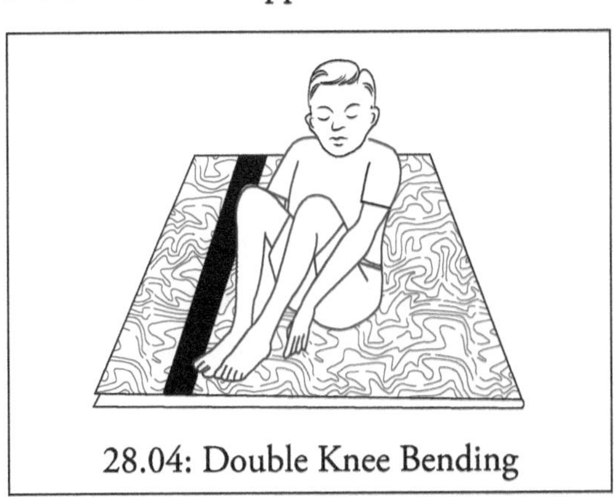

28.04: Double Knee Bending

3. Try to keep the head and spine upright. Remain in the position for a few seconds. Bend the knees and bring the legs back to the starting position, keeping the heels slightly above the floor. Draw the toes back towards the shins.

4. This is one round. Practise five to ten rounds, keeping the heels off the floor throughout the practice. The Hindi name is 'DWI JANU NAMAN.'

5. **Breathing:** Inhale while straightening the legs. Exhale while bending the legs.

6. **Focus: Mind:** On the breath, mentally counting, movements and balance.

7. Note: The hands may also be clasped under the thighs as in 'Janunaman' (Exercise Number. 28.02).

Exercise Number 28.04: THE KNEE ROTATIONS EXERCISE

In this exercise lower part of leg is to be rotated, with knee joint as centre of rotation, with upper part of leg pressed close to belly, knee touching the nose.

Steps:

1. Perform Step Number 1 to 3 of Exercise Number 28.02 (The knee movement exercise). Reach a position of knee as close to nose as feasible with support of hand grip placed below thigh.

2. Now remaining in this posture rotate the lower portion of right leg, with right knee acting as the centre of rotation. Eyes focussed on the toe. Toes pointed. Let the toe draw a circle as big as possible and as close to a circular shape as possible. Imagine that the toe is holding a brush and is painting a circle on the imaginary canvass placed vertically in front. This is also called as 'JANU CHAKRA' or 'GHOOTNA GHOOMANA.'

28.05: Knee Rotations

3. Perform ten to twelve rotations with right leg. Repeat for ten to twelve rotations of left leg.

4. **Breathing:** To be synchronised with leg rotation, inhale when leg goes up and completing the half circle upwards. Exhale when leg is coming down and completing the lower half circle. One rotation completing with one breath.

5. **Focus:** On the breath, mentally counting rotations. Eyes focussed on the toe and carefully observing the circle and the beauty of the painting on an imaginary canvass.

Exercise Number 28.05: THE ANKLE CRANK EXERCISE

Steps:

1. Remain in the starting (base) position. Bend the right knee and bring the foot towards the buttock. Turn the knee out to the side and place the foot on the left thigh. Make sure the ankle is far enough over the thigh to be free for rotation.

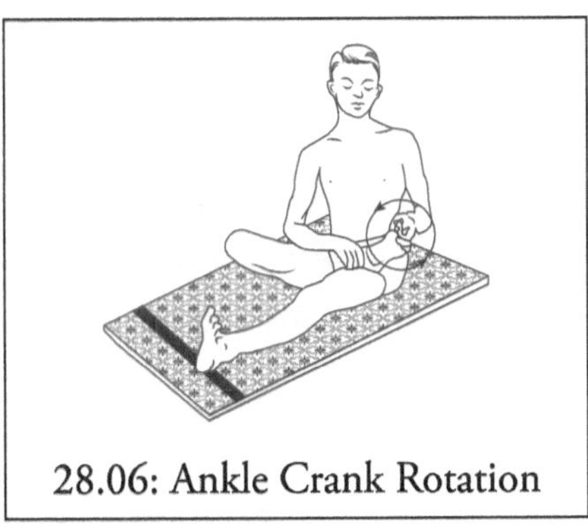

28.06: Ankle Crank Rotation

2. Hold the right ankle with the right hand to support the ankle. Hold the toes of the right foot with the left hand. A firmer grip of right foot can be achieved by inserting fingers of left hand between the toes of right foot and firmly gripping the big toe. With the aid of the left hand, slowly rotate the right foot ten to twelve times clockwise, then ten to twelve times anti-clockwise.

3. Now with left hand gripping the right foot, take your right hand on the right knee. By placing hand around the knee form a firm grip over the knee to ensure it remains stationary and stable.

4. Repeat with the left foot placed on the right thigh.

5. **Breathing:** Inhale on the upward movement of foot. Exhale on the downward movement.

6. **Focus: Mind:** On the breath, mentally counting the foot rotations. Eyes: Preferably closed or focussed on the toe.

7. **Benefits:** All the foot and calf Asanas help in returning the stagnant lymph and venous blood. They thus relieve tiredness and cramps, and prevent venous thrombosis especially in bedridden, post-operative patients. This is also called as 'GOOLF GHOORNAN.'

Exercise Number 28.06: THE HIP ROTATION EXERCISE

Steps:

1. Sit in the same starting position as for Exercise Number 28.04 above with the right leg on the left thigh.

2. Using the muscles of the right arm, rotate the right knee in a circle trying to make the smooth, jerk-free circular movement as large as possible. The index finger may be pointed out and used as a guide for observing perfections of the circular movement. Practise ten to twelve rotations clockwise and then ten to twelve rotations anti-clockwise.

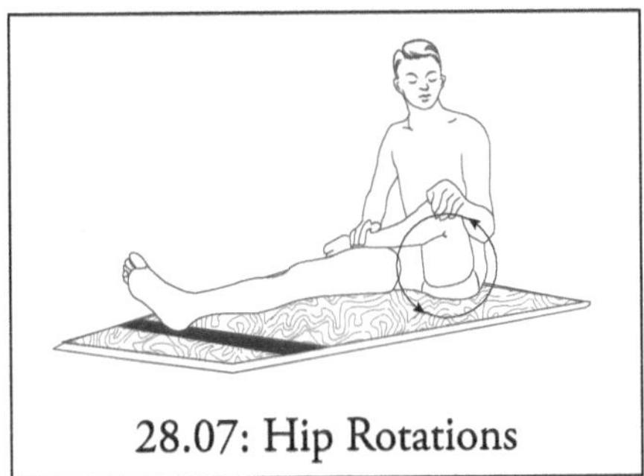

28.07: Hip Rotations

3. Straighten the leg slowly. To unlock the leg after completing Step 2, slowly and carefully straighten the leg. Bend it once, bringing the heel near the buttock. Straighten the leg. This procedure will ensure that the knee joint is realigned correctly. Release the knee by de-stretching. Repeat the same procedure with the left leg. This is called 'SHRONI CHAKRA.'

4. **Breathing:** Inhale on the upward movement of rotating leg. Exhale on the downward movement.

5. **Focus: Mind:** On the breathing, mentally counting the rotations of the hip joint and breathings. Eyes: Preferably closed or focussed on the rotational movement of knee or on tip of index finger, if kept protruding out.

Exercise Number 28.07: THE HALF BUTTERFLY POSE

Steps:

1. Sit in the starting (base) position. Bend the right leg and place the right foot as far up on the left thigh as possible. Place the right hand on top of the bent right knee. Hold the toes of the right foot with the left hand. This is the starting position, i.e., the stage I.

2. **First Variation:** (With breath synchronisation), While breathing in, gently move the right knee upwards towards the chest. Breathing out, gently push the knee down and try to touch

the knee to the floor. (See 28.08). The trunk should not move appreciably. Do not force this movement in any way. The leg muscles should be passive and loose, the movement being achieved by the exertion of force of the right arm. Slowly practise ten to twelve up and down movements. This is 'ARDHA TITALI ASANA.'

3. **Focus:** On the breath, mentally counting movement of hip joint and relaxation of inner thigh muscles.

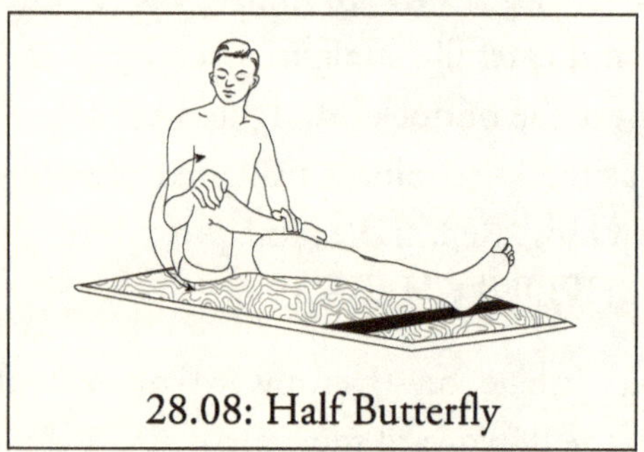

28.08: Half Butterfly

4. **Second Variation:** (Without breath synchronisation) Remain in the same position with the right leg on the left thigh. Relax the right leg muscles as much as possible. Push the right knee down with the right hand and try to touch the knee to the floor. Do not strain. Let the knee spring up by itself. The movement is achieved by use of the right arm only. Practise ten to twelve up and down movements in quick succession.

5. **Breathing:** Should be normal and unrelated to the practice. Repeat complete routine and the unwinding/unlocking procedure (see note below) with the left leg.

6. **Focus:** On mental counting, movement of hip joint and relaxation of inner thigh muscles.

7. **Note:** For unwinding/unlocking: To unlock the leg after completing exercise routine, slowly and carefully straighten the leg. Bend it once, bringing the heel near the buttock.

Straighten the leg. This procedure will ensure that the knee joint is realigned correctly

Exercise Number 28.08: THE FULL BUTTERFLY POSE

Precautions:

Persons suffering from sciatica and sacral conditions should not practice this Asana.

Steps:

1. Sit in the base position. Bend the knees and bring the sole of the feet together, keeping the heels as close to the body as possible. Heels may be as close to the reproductive organ as comfortable. Fully relax the inner thigh muscles.

2. **Variation 1:** Clasp the feet with both hands. Gently bounce the knees up and down, using the elbows as levers to press the legs down. (See 28.09). Try to touch the knees to the ground on the downward stroke. Do not use any force. Practise twenty to thirty up and down movements. These up and down movements of the leg should be as smooth as the movements of the wings of a flying butterfly. The asana derives its name from butterfly wings and is called as 'POORNA-TITALI-ASANA.'

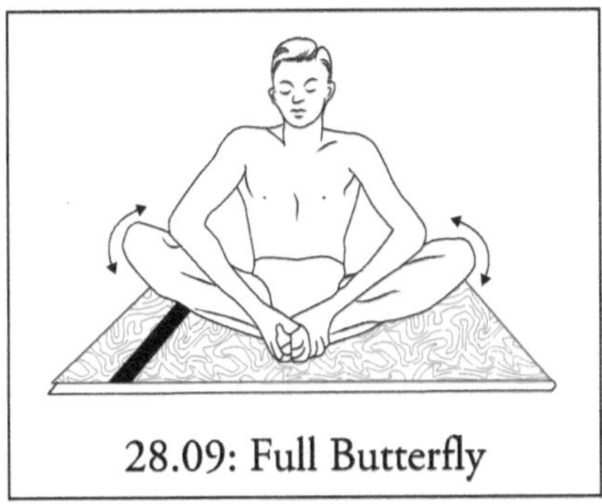

28.09: Full Butterfly

3. **Variation 2:** Keep the soles of the feet together. Place the hands on the knees. Using the palms, gently push the knees down towards

the floor, allowing them to spring up again all by themselves. (See 28.10) Do not force this movement. Repeat twenty to thirty times. Straighten the legs and relax.

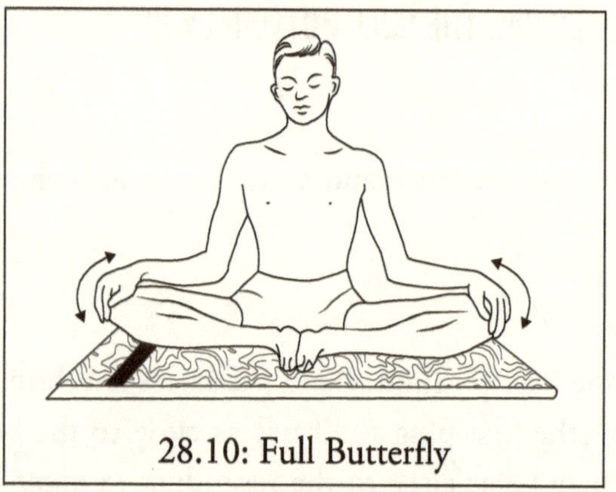

28.10: Full Butterfly

4. **Breathing:** Normal breathing, unrelated to the practice.

5. **Focus: Mind:** On mental counting, movement and relaxation. Eyes: Closed.

Day Twenty-Nine: The Subtle Exercises for Hands: Part – I

Having learnt to take good care of our legs, we have now earned our first promotion. We have moved up in life. The focus of our attention now is our hands. So! Let's take good care of them too.

Learning and Practices for the Day

Exercise Number 29.01: THE HAND CLENCHING EXERCISE

Steps:

1. Sit in the Prarambhikstithi (i.e., the base position) or a cross-legged (e.g., Sukhasana) pose.

2. Hold both arms straight in front of the body at shoulder level. Open the hands, palms down, and stretch the fingers as wide apart as possible.

3. Close the fingers to make a tight fist with the thumbs inside. The fingers should be slowly wrapped around the thumbs. (See 29.01) Again, open the hands and stretch the fingers. Repeat ten to twelve times. Feel the stretching of muscles from shoulder joints to fingertips.

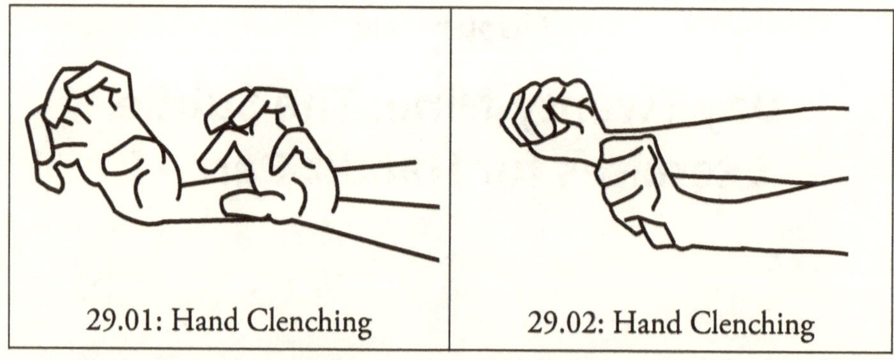

| 29.01: Hand Clenching | 29.02: Hand Clenching |

4. Now close the fingers to make a tight fist with the thumbs outside. The fingers should be slowly wrapped to touch the bottom most points in palms, and thumbs should press the index fingers at their bases. (See 29.02).

5. Again, open the hands and stretch the fingers. Repeat ten to twelve times. This is also named as 'MUSHTIKA BANDHANA.' 'Mushtika' and 'Mutthi' are Sanskrit words for fist.

6. **Breathing:** Inhale on opening the hands. Exhale on closing the hands.

7. **Focus: Mind:** Focussed on the breath, mentally counting, stretching sensation and movements. Eyes: Closed or focussed on fist.

Exercise Number 29.02: THE WRIST BENDING EXERCISE

Steps:

1. Remain in the base position or a cross-legged pose. Stretch the arms in front of the body at shoulder level. Keep the palms open and fingers straight throughout the entire exercise.

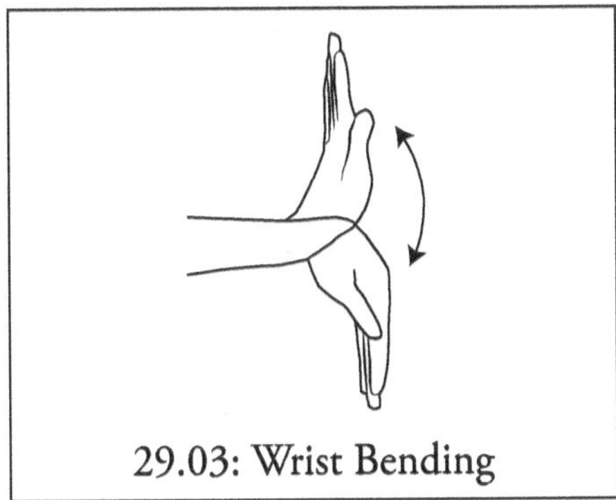

29.03: Wrist Bending

2. Bend the hands backwards from the wrists, as if pressing the palms against a wall with the fingers pointing towards the ceiling or sky. Now, bend the hands forward from the wrists so that the fingers point towards the floor.

3. Keep the elbows straight throughout the practice. Do not bend the knuckle joints or fingers. Bend the hands up again for the next round. Repeat ten to twelve times. This is 'MANIBANDHA NAMAN.'

4. **Breathing:** Inhale with the upward movements. Exhale with the downward movements.

5. **Focus: Mind:** On the breath, mentally counting the breathings and the movements. Eyes: Closed or focussed on fingertips or wrists.

Exercise Number 29.03: **THE WRIST JOINT ROTATION EXERCISE**

Steps:

1. Remain in the base position or a comfortable cross-legged pose but keep the spine and back straight.

2. **Phase 1:** Extend the right arm forward at shoulder level. Make a fist with the right hand, with the thumb inside. The left hand may be used as a support to hold the elbow, if necessary. This is the starting position. Slowly rotate the fist around the wrist, ensuring that the palm faces downward throughout the rotation. The arms and elbows should remain perfectly straight and still. Make as large a circle as possible. (See 29.04)

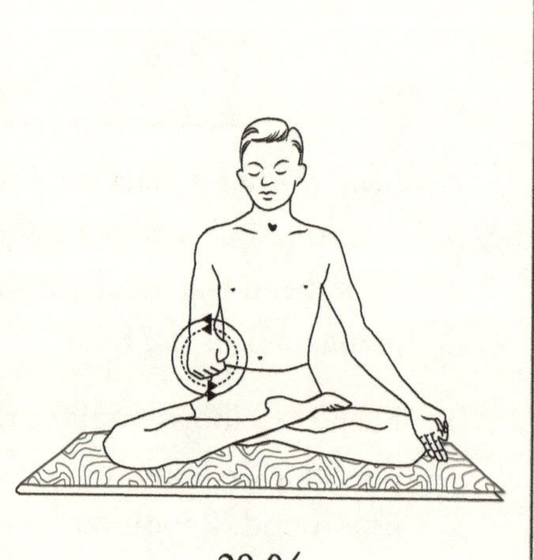

29.04

3. Feel the rotations of the groups of muscles between shoulder joint and palm. Practise ten to twelve times clockwise and ten to twelve times anti-clockwise. Repeat the same with the left fist.

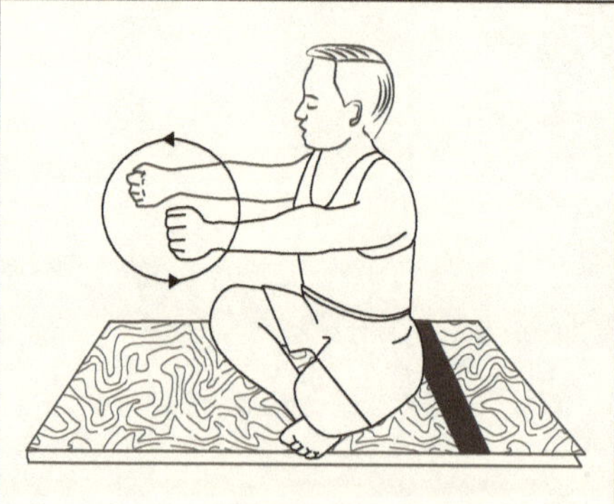

29.05

4. **Phase 2:** Extend both arms in front of the body with the fists clenched. Keep the arms straight and at shoulder level. Rotate both the fists together in the same direction. Practise ten to twelve times in each direction. (See 29.05)

5. **Phase 3:** Practise as in Phase 2. Rotate the fists together in the opposite directions, i.e., left fist clockwise and right fist anti-clockwise and vice-versa. Practise ten to twelve times in each direction. (See 29.06) You are performing 'MANIBANDHA CHAKRA'

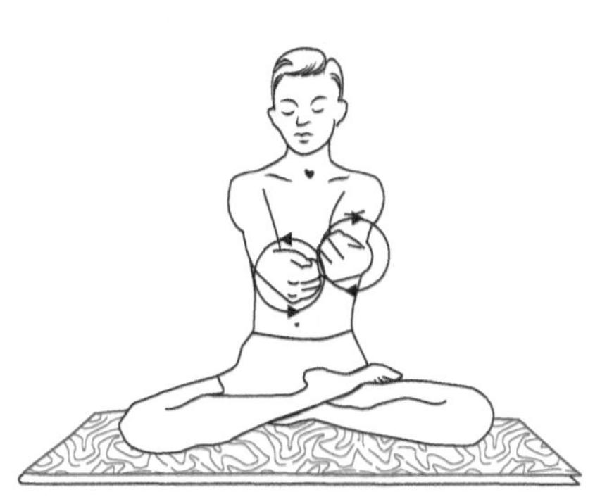

29.06

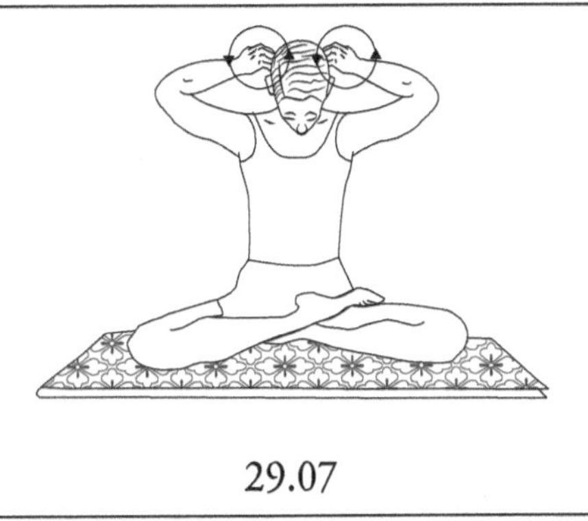

29.07

6. **Phase 4:** In this exercise fists, tightly clenched, are to be rotated around the ears. The fists shall make a circular motion, with centre point of ears acting as the centre point of rotation. (See 29.07)

7. Left fist to be rotated around left ear and right fist around right ear. Elbows will remain pointing outwards, the upper arm remaining parallel to the ground. Complete ten to twelve swift rotations in clockwise direction and equal numbers of rotations in anti-clockwise direction, with breath synchronisations.

8. **Breathing:** Normal, unrelated to the movements, but synchronised with rotations, i.e., one rotation corresponding to one breath. Exhale when the fist is at the bottommost point in the circular motion. This way breath synchronisation can be smoothly achieved.

9. **Focus: Mind:** On the breath, mentally counting the breathings and rotations. Eyes: Preferably closed or focussed on fist observing the smoothness of circular motion and guiding the fist(s).

Exercise Number 29.04: THE ELBOW BENDING EXERCISE

Steps:

1. **Phase – 1:** Remain in the base position or a cross-legged pose. Stretch the arms in front of the body at shoulder level. The hands should be open with the palms facing up. Bend the arms at the elbows and touch the fingers to the shoulders. Straighten the arms again. This is one round. Repeat ten to twelve times.

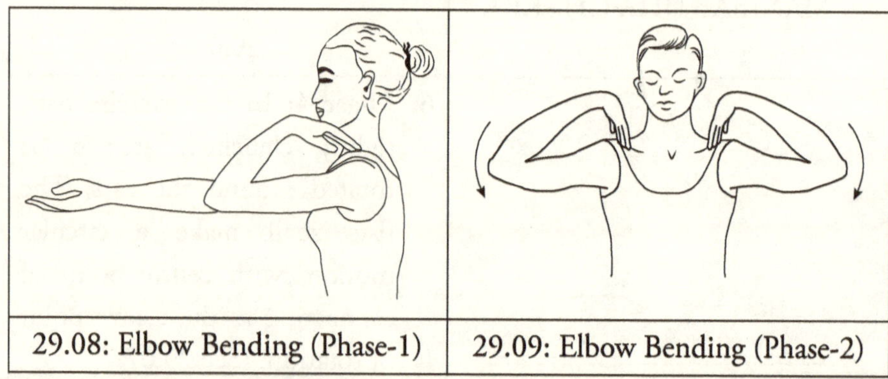

29.08: Elbow Bending (Phase-1)	29.09: Elbow Bending (Phase-2)

2. **Phase – 2:** Extend the arms sideways at shoulder level, hands open and palms facing the ceiling or sky. Bend the arms at the elbows and touch the fingers to the shoulders. Again, straighten the arms sideways. Repeat ten to twelve times. This is 'KEHUNI NAMAN.'

3. **Breathing:** Inhale while straightening the arms. Exhale while bending the arms.

4. **Focus: Mind:** On the breathing, mentally counting the movements. Eyes: Preferably closed or focussed on arms movements, following and guiding the movements.

5. **Note:** Throughout both stages, the upper arms remain parallel to the floor, and elbows remain at shoulder level.

Chapter–Four

Day-Thirty: The Subtle Exercises for Hands: Part – II

Learning and Practice for the Day

Perform all exercises in this series in smooth progression of exercises in previous series.

Exercise Number 30.01: THE ARMS ROTATION EXERCISE

Steps:

1. Remain in the base position or a cross-legged pose. Loosen the arms and form close, tight fists with both hands. Allow hands, hinged on shoulders, to be bent at elbows, making an angle of 90 degrees at elbow joints, fist pointed in front directions.

2. From this posture, take your hand forcefully up, making a swift motion, fist remaining closed, take hands over the head and in backward direction as far as possible. Elbows shall remain at 90 degrees. As soon as the hands reach the peak point, behind the back, again bring them down and take elbows backwards as far as possible. All motions should be smooth but swift and fast. The shoulder socket will get lubricated, strengthened and rejuvenated.

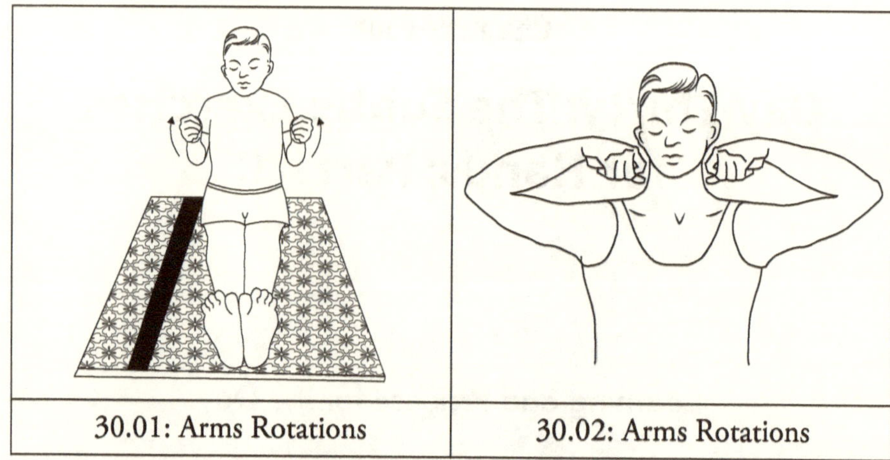

| 30.01: Arms Rotations | 30.02: Arms Rotations |

3. Rotate the arms on the axis of your shoulder, the pivot point of shoulder and arms experiencing a swift rotation.

4. One up and down movement is one round. Repeat ten to twelve times. In Hindi, you were doing 'HAATH GOOMANA.'

5. **Breathing:** Inhale while taking the arms up and fists backwards. Exhale while arms are coming down and elbows going backwards. Inhale and exhale forcefully to allow the power of your lungs help in rotational movements around the shoulder.

6. **Focus:** On the breathing, mentally counting the movements.

7. **Note:** During the rotational movements, lower part of arms should remain parallel to the floor, when crossing the central point of rotation. Upper portion of arms should at least become parallel to surface, when they reach the peak point at the top.

Exercise Number 30.02: SHOULDER SOCKET ROTATION, WITH HANDS AT COLLAR BONES

Steps:

1. Immediately after completing the Exercise Number 30.01 and as soon as breathing becomes normal, join all fingers and thumbs

of both hands separately, such that all tips are joined in the same plane forming a circular shape.

2. Place the fingers of the left hand on the left side of collar bone and the fingers of the right hand on the right side of collar bone. Fully rotate both elbows at the same time in a large circle, keeping both hands firmly touching the collarbones.

3. Try to touch the elbows in front of the chest on the forward movement and touch the ears while moving up. Stretch the arms back in the backward movement and touch the sides of the trunk while coming down. Practise slowly ten to twelve times clockwise and then ten to twelve times anti-clockwise.

4. Fingers and thumbs should remain joined together and firmly placed on respective collar bones. Tips of fingers of both hands should be touching each other or be a few millimetres apart.

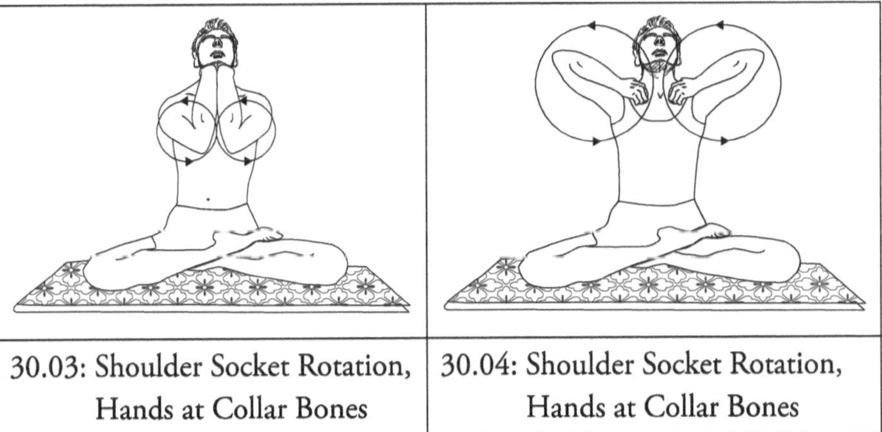

30.03: Shoulder Socket Rotation, Hands at Collar Bones	30.04: Shoulder Socket Rotation, Hands at Collar Bones

5. **Breathing:** Inhale on the upward stroke. Exhale on the downward stroke.

6. **Focus:** On the breath, mentally counting the rotations focussed on the stretching sensation around the shoulder joint.

Exercise Number 30.03: THE SHOULDER SOCKET ROTATION EXERCISE

Steps:

1. Remain in the base position or a cross-legged pose.

2. **Phase – 1:** Place the fingers (joined together, finger tips in the same plane, circular shape) of the right hand on the right shoulder. Keep the left hand on the left knee in Jnana mudra and the back straight. Rotate the right elbow in a large circle. Practise ten to twelve times clockwise and ten to twelve times anti-clockwise. Repeat with the left elbow. Make sure that the head, trunk and spine remain straight and still.

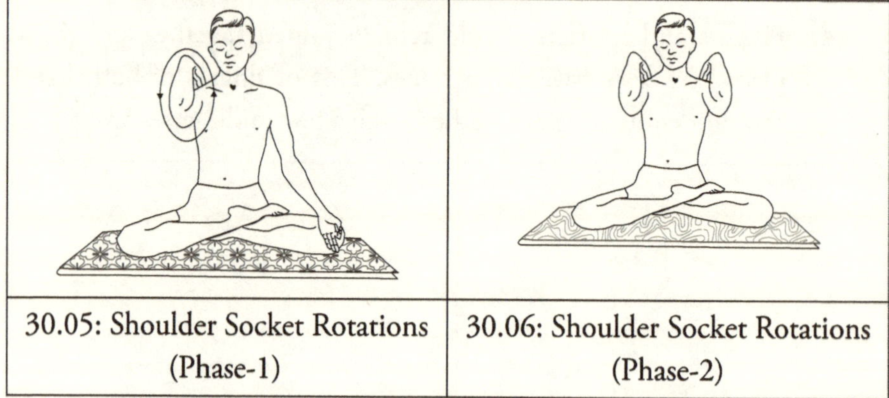

30.05: Shoulder Socket Rotations (Phase-1)	30.06: Shoulder Socket Rotations (Phase-2)

3. **Phase – 2:** Place the fingers of the left hand on the left shoulder and the fingers of the right hand on the right shoulder. Fully rotate both elbows at the same time in a large circle. Try to touch the elbows in front of the chest on the forward movement and touch the ears while moving up. Stretch the arms back in the backward movement and touch the sides of the trunk while coming down. Allow the skin of your arms to gently massage your face in each circular motion. This will bring glow to your face. Do not bother about the sweating. If slightly wet arms are massaging the face, it is better. Practise slowly ten to twelve times

clockwise and then ten to twelve times anti-clockwise. This was 'SKANDHA CHAKRA.'

4. **Breathing:** Inhale on the upward stroke. Exhale on the downward stroke.

5. **Focus: Mind:** On the breath, mentally counting and feeling the stretching sensation around the shoulder joint. Eyes: Shut.

6. **Benefits:** This exercise relieves the strain of driving and office work and is helpful in cervical spondylitis and frozen shoulder. This also maintains the shape of the shoulders and chest.

Day Thirty-One: The Subtle Exercises for Neck

Hey! Congratulations on the next promotion. We shall now be focussing our energies on the neck.

Learning and Practice for the Day

Exercise Number 31.01: THE NECK MOVEMENTS EXERCISE

Precautions:

This exercise involves some very sensitive and delicate parts of your body. Though on the face of it, the exercise looks very simple and harmless, all the muscles and nerves connecting your brain to all other organs are involved, one way or the other.

So, abundant precautions are required. No jerks and no overstretching are the guiding mantras. These four neck movements should not be performed by elderly people and those suffering from low blood pressure, very high blood pressure, extreme cervical spondylitis or any other nerves related disorders.

The advice of an expert should be sought for any of these problems. Patients of cervical spondylitis should strictly avoid forward bending of the neck.

Steps:

1. **Phase – 1**: Sit in the base position or a cross-legged pose with the hands resting on the knees in 'Jnana Mudra.' Close the eyes.

Slowly move the head forward and try to touch the chin to the chest. Now move the head as far back as comfortable. Do not strain. Try to feel the stretch of the muscles in the front and back of the neck, and the loosening of the vertebrae in the neck. Practise ten to twelve times.

2. **Breathing:** Inhale on the backward movement. Exhale on the forward movement.

3. **Phase – 2:** Remain in the same position, keeping the eyes closed, and face directly forward. Relax the shoulders. Slowly move the head to the right and try to touch the right ear to the right shoulder raising the shoulder. Move the head to the left side and try to touch the left ear to the left shoulder. This is one round. Do not strain; touching the ear with shoulder is not necessary, try to bring the head as close to shoulder as feasible, without jerks and without overstretching. Practise ten to twelve rounds.

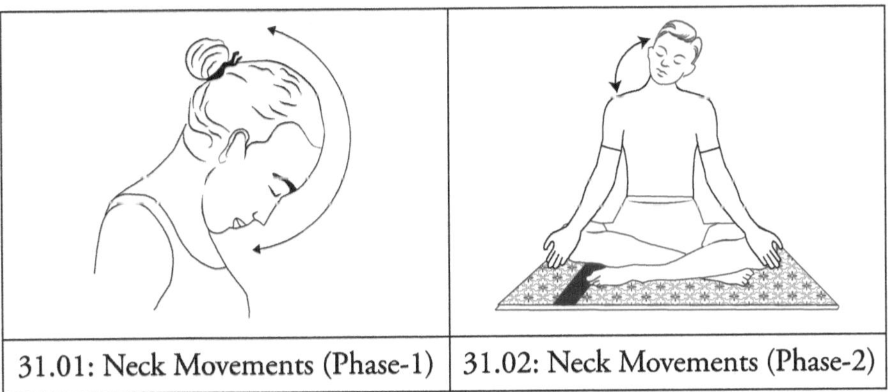

| 31.01: Neck Movements (Phase-1) | 31.02: Neck Movements (Phase-2) |

4. **Breathing:** Inhale on the upward movement. Exhale on the downward movement.

5. **Focus:** On the breath, counting, and the stretching sensation of the muscles in the sides of the neck.

Tip of the Day

'Kapalabhati' is one of the simplest of the Pranayamas. It is easy to understand. There are very few steps to remember. It is also easy to perform. Particularly the slower version, of simply exhaling only, almost occurs naturally.

If you have started practising Pranayama routinely, one issue that you may be encountering is that you may, during practice, forget the predetermined sequence of Pranayama exercises. You may either be stuck on Kapalabhati only and keep on performing it endlessly, or in between forget the next Pranayama set out initially, and instead of next Pranayama in sequence, start performing Kapalabhati.

The easiest way to counter this problem is to use Kapalabhati as filler in the Pranayama series, i.e., set out your sequence with other Pranayamas ignoring Kapalabhati, and allow it to happen automatically, during those moments of forgetfulness.

Or alternatively, keep Kapalabhati as the last set in your sequence of Pranayama. This way, at the last you may check if you have already performed it instinctively in between. If yes, you may skip it, at the last stage.

6. **Phase – 3:** Remain in the base position. Keep the head upright and the eyes closed. Gently turn the head to the right so that the chin is in line with the shoulder. Feel the release of tension in the neck muscles and the loosening of the neck joints. Slowly turn the head to the left as far as is comfortable. Do not strain. Practise ten to twelve times on each side.

7. **Breathing:** Inhale while turning to the front. Exhale while turning to the sides.

8. **Phase – 4:** Remain in the same position with the eyes closed. Slowly rotate the head downward, to the right, backward and

then to the left side in relaxed, smooth, rhythmic, circular movements. Feel the shifting stretch around the neck and the loosening up of the joints and muscles of the neck. While rotating the head, try to touch the chin with the collarbone in the downward position and touch the ear with left and right shoulders, while crossing over the shoulders. Try to take the head as backwards as feasible. All movements must be smooth with full enjoyment. Practise ten to twelve times clockwise and then ten to twelve times anti-clockwise. Do not strain. 'GREEVA SANCHALANA' is the Hindi name.

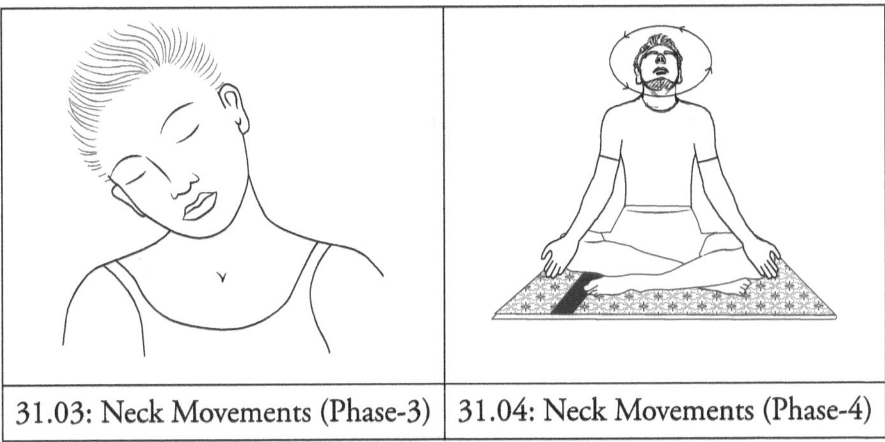

| 31.03: Neck Movements (Phase-3) | 31.04: Neck Movements (Phase-4) |

9. If dizziness occurs, open the eyes. After the practice, keep the neck straight and the eyes closed. Be aware of the sensations in the head and neck.

10. **Breathing:** Inhale as the head moves up. Exhale as the head moves down.

11. **Focus:** On the breath, mentally counting the rotations and breathings.

Day Thirty-Two: The Subtle Exercises in Lying down Postures: Part – I

Learning and Practice for the Day

The exercises in this series strengthen the abdominal muscles and massage the organs connected with digestion systems. They strengthen the digestive system, lower back, pelvic and perineal muscles and helps correct prolapse. These exercises are good for hip and knee joints. All exercises of this series are also recommended to be performed in sequential manner, as narrated. The salient benefits of exercises in this series are:

- Strengthens abdominal and lower back muscles, loosens the vertebrae.

- Some exercises are effective in removing wind and constipation.

- By massaging the pelvic muscles and reproductive organs, they are also useful in the treatment of impotency, sterility and menstrual problems.

- Some subtle postures massage the back, buttocks and hips. They are useful if done first thing in the morning after waking up.

- Some give an excellent stretch to the abdominal muscles and organs, thereby helping to improve digestion and eliminate constipation. The twisting stretch of the spinal muscles relieves the strain and stiffness caused by prolonged sitting.

- Tightness and tiredness are relieved.

- A few practices stimulate the muscular, digestive, circulatory, nervous and hormonal systems, tone all the organs and remove lethargy. They are especially useful for eliminating nervous tension and bringing about deep relaxation.

Exercise Number 32.01: BOTH LEGS SLIGHTLY RAISED UP POSTURE

Steps:

1. Lie down flat on your back in the starting or relaxation posture of Shavasana (Supine Posture-Base position) with hands by the sides of body and the palms flat on the floor.

2. **Phase – 1:** Inhale deeply and raise both the legs, slightly above the ground, just ten to fifteen centimetres. Keep the legs straight, toes pointed and the feet relaxed. The leg-line and spine-line should be making an obtuse angle of slightly less than 180 degrees, i.e., legs raised up at an angle of about five to ten degrees only above the ground surface. Do not allow your head to rise. Hold the posture for fifteen to twenty seconds, counting mentally and retaining the breath.

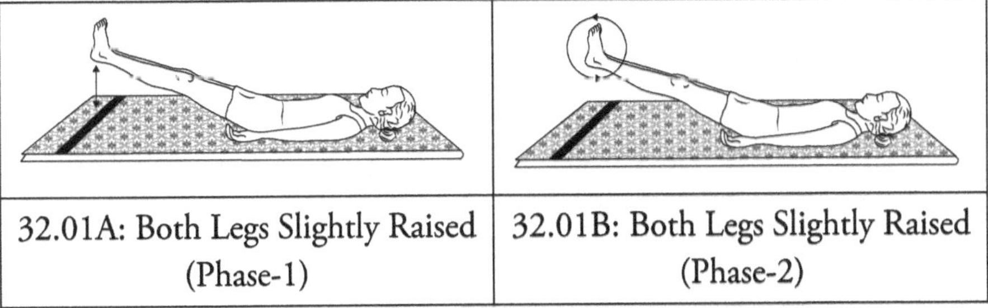

32.01A: Both Legs Slightly Raised (Phase-1)	32.01B: Both Legs Slightly Raised (Phase-2)

3. Exhale normally and slowly lower the legs to the floor. This is one round. Practise two to four rounds. This asana is called 'UTTHAN PADASANA.'

4. **Breathing:** Inhale while raising the legs. Hold the posture and retain the breath. Exhale while lowering the legs.

5. **Focus:** Mind: Focussed on synchronising the movement with the breath, the stretch in the legs, compression in belly region and mentally counting in the final position. Eyes: Preferably closed, if open focussed on a point in the ceiling or sky.

6. **Phase – 2:** Raise both the legs, joined together, by ten to fifteen centimetres above the ground, big toes touching each other. Rotate both legs in circles of very small diameter. Head and back shall be firmly resting on ground. Maintain breath synchronisation of one breath for one rotation. Rotate five to six times in clockwise direction and five to six times in anti-clockwise direction. Lower the legs and relax.

7. **Note:** This is the warming up routine. It will warm up your body and prepare it for subsequent exercises in this section. Practise it first and thereafter only attempt the rest of the exercises. Do not ignore it, howsoever innocent or easy it may appear to you, initially.

Exercise Number 32.02: THE RAISED LEGS POSTURE

Steps:

1. Lie in the starting position of Shavasana posture (Supine Posture-Base position) with the palms flat on the floor. Inhale and raise the right leg as high as comfortable, keeping it straight, toes pointed and the foot relaxed.

2. Try to bring the leg up in truly vertical position, i.e., the leg-line and spine-line making an angle close to 90 degrees. The left leg should remain straight and in contact with the floor. Hold the posture for three to five seconds, counting mentally and retaining the breath.

3. Exhale and slowly lower the leg to the floor. This is one round. Practise five to six rounds with the right leg and then five to six rounds with the left leg.

4. This is to be followed by raising both legs together, holding the legs raised posture for three to five seconds for five to six repetitions.

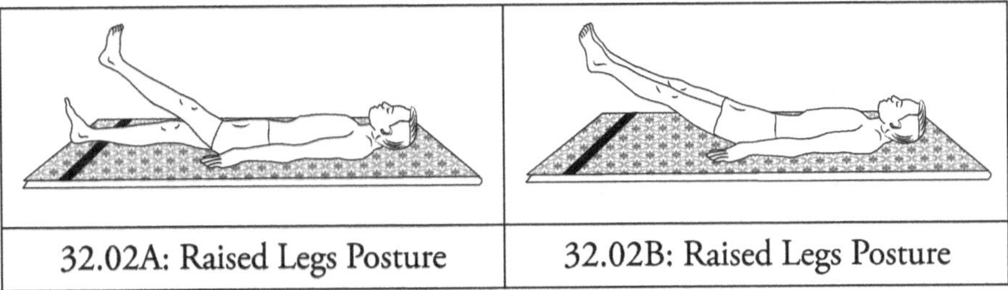

| 32.02A: Raised Legs Posture | 32.02B: Raised Legs Posture |

5. **Breathing:** Inhale: While raising the leg or legs. Hold the posture and retain the breath. Exhale: While lowering the leg or legs.

6. **Focus:** Mind: Focussed on synchronising the movement with the breath, the stretch in the legs and mentally counting in the final position. Eyes: Preferably closed, if open focussed on the toe(s) of leg(s) being lifted.

7. **Note:** If raising legs by 90 degrees is difficult initially, raised leg poses may be repeated raising the legs to progressive heights of 15, 25, 35, 45 cm respectively in each round.

Exercise Number 32.03: THE LEG ROTATIONS EXERCISE

Steps:

1. Lie down in the starting posture of Shavasana (Supine Posture-Base position). Keep the arms by the sides of trunk, palms facing upwards.

2. **Phase – 1:** Raise the right leg 5 cm from the ground, keeping the knee straight. Rotate the entire leg clockwise ten to twelve times in as large a circle as possible. The heel should not touch the floor at any time during the rotation. Toes to remain pointed. Rotate ten to twelve times in the opposite direction. Repeat equal number of rotations in both directions with the left leg. Do not strain.

3. Rest in the relaxation posture (base position) introducing abdominal breathing until the respiration returns to normal.

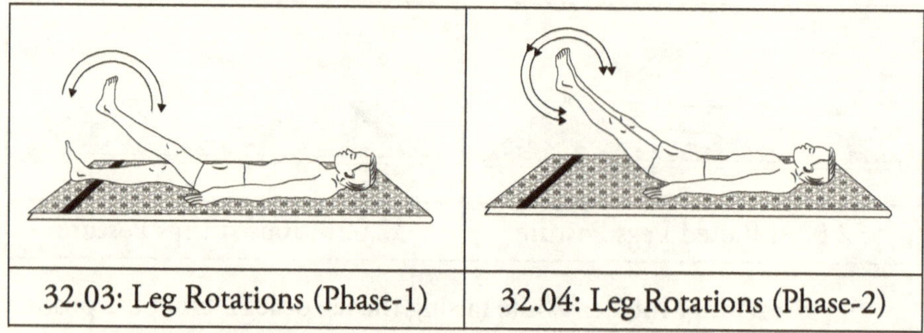

| 32.03: Leg Rotations (Phase-1) | 32.04: Leg Rotations (Phase-2) |

4. **Phase – 2:** Raise both legs together. Keep them together and straight throughout the practice, big toes pointed and touching each other. Rotate both legs clockwise and then anti-clockwise three to five times. The circular movement should be as smooth and as large as possible. Imagine drawing up a circle on an imaginary canvas placed vertically, with the brush firmly held between the big toes.

5. **Breathing:** Breathe normally throughout the practice.

6. **Focus:** Mind: Focussed on the mental counting of each round, rotation of the leg(s) and on the effects of the asana on the hips and abdomen areas. Eyes: Preferably closed, if open, focussed on the toe(s) of leg(s) being rotated, tracing the full rotation and guiding the leg in making the motion in perfectly circular manner.

Day Thirty-Three: The Subtle Exercises in Lying down Postures: Part – II

Learning and Practice for the Day

Perform exercises in this series also in the manner of smooth progression after completing all or at least a few of the exercises of previous series.

Exercise Number 33.01: THE YOGIC CYCLING (PADA SANCHALANASANA)

Steps:

1. Lie in the starting position of Shavasana (Supine Posture-Base position).

2. **Phase – 1:** (Pedalling the cycle with one leg): Raise the right leg. Bend the knee and bring the thigh to the chest. Raise and straighten the leg completely.

3. Then, lower the straight leg in a forward movement. Bend the knee and bring it back to the chest to complete the cycling movement. The heel should not touch the floor during the movement. Toes pointed. Repeat ten to twelve times in a forward direction and then ten to twelve times in reverse. Repeat with the left leg.

4. **Breathing:** Inhale while straightening the leg. Exhale while bending the knee and bringing the thigh to the chest.

5. **Phase – 2:** (Pedalling the cycle with both legs) Raise both legs. Practise alternate cycling movements as though pedalling

a bicycle. Practise ten to twelve times forward and then ten to twelve times backwards.

6. **Breathing:** Breathe normally throughout.

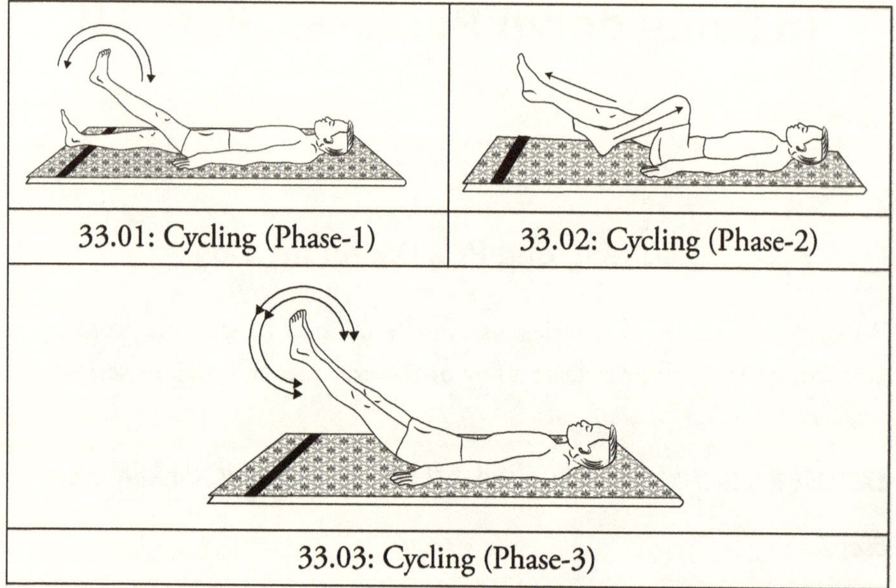

| 33.01: Cycling (Phase-1) | 33.02: Cycling (Phase-2) |

33.03: Cycling (Phase-3)

7. **Phase – 3:** Raise both legs and keep them together throughout the practice. Toes pointed and touching. Bring the knees as close as possible to the chest on the backward movement and straighten the legs fully on the forward movement. Slowly lower the legs together, keeping the knees straight, until the legs are just above the floor. Then bend the knees and bring them back to the chest. Practise three to five forward cycling movements and the same in reverse. Do not strain.

8. **Breathing:** Inhale while straightening the legs. Exhale while bending the legs to the chest.

9. **Focus: Mind:** Focussed on the breath, mental counting of each round and on smoothness of the movement and proper coordination, especially while reverse cycling. When relaxing, be aware of the abdomen, hip, thighs and lower back. **Eyes:** Preferably closed;

if open, pointedly focussed on the moving organs (Knee, Toe), tracing the full movement and guiding the organ in making the motion in the prescribed manner.

10. **Note:** Keep the rest of the body, including the head, flat on the ground throughout the practice. After completing each stage remain in the base position and relax until breathing becomes normal. If cramping is experienced in the abdominal muscles, inhale deeply, gently pushing out the abdomen, and then relax the whole body with exhalation.

11. Do not strain, this applies especially to Phase-3. Phase-3 is strenuous, practise it carefully.

Exercise Number 33.02: THE SLEEPING WIND RELEASING POSTURE (LEG LOCK POSE)

Precautions:

This exercise is not to be performed by persons suffering from high blood pressure or serious back conditions, such as sciatica and slipped disc. Those having back pains may practise very, very slowly, and without lifting the head, under medical/experts' supervision.

Steps:

1. Lie down flat on the back (Supine Posture-Base position).

2. **Phase – 1:** Bend the right knee and bring the thigh to the chest. Interlock the fingers, inserting the fingers in right hand, between the gaps in fingers of left hand alternatively, thus locking both hands together. Keeping palms in front, clasp the hands on the shin just below the right knee. Keep the left leg straight and on the ground. Inhale deeply, filling the lungs with as much air as possible. Holding the breath, raise the head and shoulders off the ground and try to touch the right knee with the nose.

3. Remain in the final position for a few seconds, retaining the breath and counting mentally. While slowly exhaling, return to the base position. Relax the body. Repeat three times with the right leg and then three times with the left leg.

4. **Note:** Ensure that the straight leg remains in contact with the ground. It is important to start with the right leg because it presses the ascending colon directly. Follow with the left leg which presses the descending colon directly.

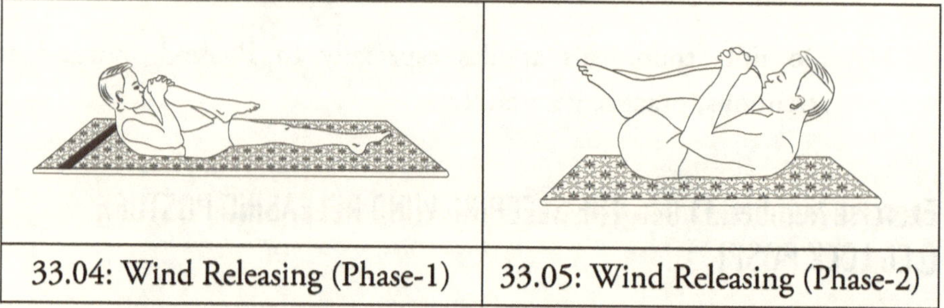

| 33.04: Wind Releasing (Phase-1) | 33.05: Wind Releasing (Phase-2) |

5. **Phase – 2:** Remain in the base position. Bend both knees and bring the thighs to the chest. Interlock the fingers and clasp the hands on the shin bones just below the knees. Inhale deeply. Holding the breath, raise the head and shoulders and try to place the nose in the space between the two knees. Keep toes pointed throughout the practice. Hold the breath in the raised position for a few seconds, counting mentally. Slowly lower the head, shoulders and legs while breathing out. Practise these three times. The Hindi name of this posture is 'SUPTA PAWAN MUKT ASANA' meaning 'the wind releasing posture in sleeping mode.'

6. **Focus:** Mind: Focussed on the breath, mentally counting in the final position, pressure on the abdomen and the movement.

7. **Variants:** Repeat the practice as described in Phase 1 and 2 but change the breathing pattern slightly. Instead of inhaling before raising the body, exhale deeply and hold the breath out in the final position for a few seconds, counting mentally. Lower the head,

shoulders and leg(s) while breathing in. Practise three rounds for both Phases 1 and 2.

Exercise Number 33.03: YOGIC ROCK and ROLLS

Precautions:

Not to be performed by persons with serious back conditions, back pain, or suffering from any spine related diseases.

Steps:

1. Lie down flat on the back (Supine Posture-Base position).

2. **Phase – 1:** Bend both legs to the chest. Interlock the fingers of both hands and clasp them around the shins just below the knees. Keep your nose in between the knees or as close as comfortably possible. Keep toes pointed. This is the starting position. Roll the complete body from side to side, keeping spine as the centre of rotation five to ten times, touching the side of the legs on the floor. Try to touch the ground with your nose when the body is in extreme left or right side. If touching ground with nose is difficult, the knees must kiss the ground.

3. **Breathing:** Breathe normally throughout.

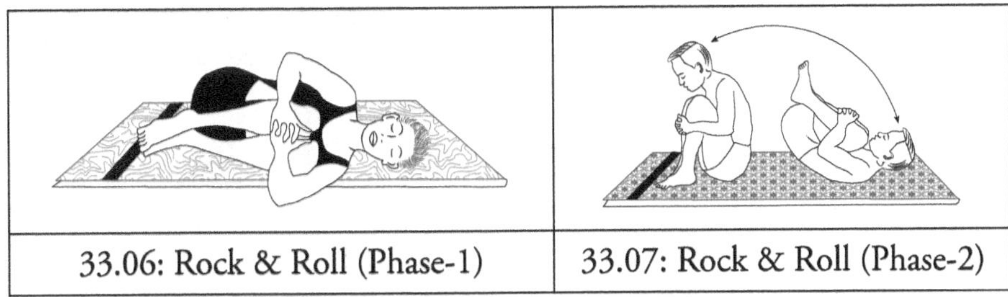

| 33.06: Rock & Roll (Phase-1) | 33.07: Rock & Roll (Phase-2) |

4. **Phase – 2:** Sit in the squatting position with the buttocks just above the floor. Interlock the fingers of both hands and clasp them around the shins just below the knees. Rock the whole body backwards and forwards on the spine, keeping your hips as

central point of rotation. Try to come up into the squatting pose on the feet when rocking forward. If it is difficult to perform with the hands clasped on the shins, then hold the sides of the thighs adjacent to the knees. Practise five to ten backward and forward movements.

5. **Breathing:** Breathe normally throughout.

6. **Focus:** Mind: Focussed on the coordination of movement. While relaxing in Shavasana be aware of the effects of the asana on the back and buttocks. Eyes: Preferably closed, if open focussed on one point at centre of knees.

7. **Note:** Use a folded blanket for this practice so that there is no possibility of causing damage to the spine. While rocking back, the head should remain forward. Be careful not to hit the head on the floor. The posture is also called as 'JHULANA LURHAKANA ASANA' meaning 'Swinging' and 'back and forth movements' respectively.

Exercise Number 33.04: SLEEPING ABDOMINAL STRETCH POSE: (MARKATA-ASANA-1)

Precautions:

Not to be performed by persons with serious back conditions, back pain, or suffering from any spine/sciatica nerve related diseases, unless instructed by a medical practitioner/expert.

Steps:

1. Lie in the starting posture of Shavasana (Supine Posture-Base position).

2. **Phase – 1:** Bend the knees and place the soles of both feet flat on the ground, directly in front of the buttocks. Keep the knees and feet together throughout the practice. Interlock the fingers of both hands and place the palms under the back of the head.

3. While breathing out, slowly lower the legs to the right, trying to bring the knees down to the floor. The feet should remain in contact with each other, although the left foot will move slightly off the floor. At the same time, gently turn the head and neck in the opposite direction to the legs. This will give a uniform twisting stretch to the entire spine. Hold the breath in the final position while mentally counting three seconds. (See 33.08)

4. While breathing in, raise both legs to the upright position. Keep the shoulders and elbows on the floor throughout. Repeat on the left side to complete one round. Practise five to six complete rounds.

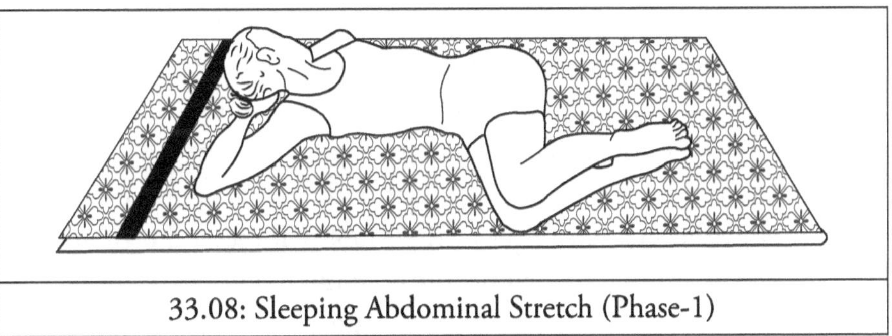

33.08: Sleeping Abdominal Stretch (Phase-1)

5. **Breathing:** Exhale while lowering the legs to the sides. Hold the breath in the final position. Inhale while raising the legs.

6. **Focus:** Mind: Focussed on the breath, the brain mentally counting, in the final position and the twisting stretch on the para-spinal and abdominal muscles.

7. **Variations:** Bend the knees and bring the thighs up to the chest. Interlock the fingers and place them behind the head. Roll the body from side to side, keeping the elbows on the floor.

8. **Phase – 2:** Practise Steps No 1 and 2 of Phase 1, by keeping feet close to buttocks, but maintain some gap (say around one foot apart). When feet are moving in right directions, the head shall move in left directions and so on. Both legs and knees shall remain

apart and away from each other, however both shall move in the same direction. Complete five to six rounds. (See 33.09)

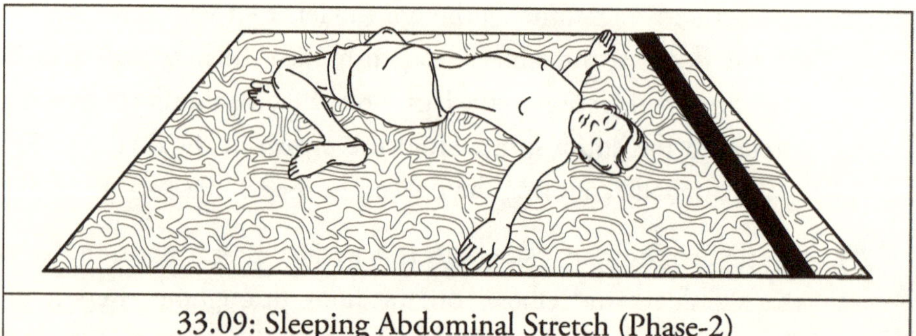

33.09: Sleeping Abdominal Stretch (Phase-2)

9. **Phase – 3:** Now stretch the legs in front. Keeping both legs on ground and maintaining around one foot distance between the two heels, bring both feet together to the left, such that the smallest finger of left foot touches the ground, the thumb of right foot also touches the ground, near the left heel. Head will go in right direction. Now, shift both feet in opposite direction. Now the smallest finger of right foot will touch the ground, the thumb of left foot will be touching the ground close to the right heel. Head will go in left, i.e., opposite to the foot direction. (See 33.10)

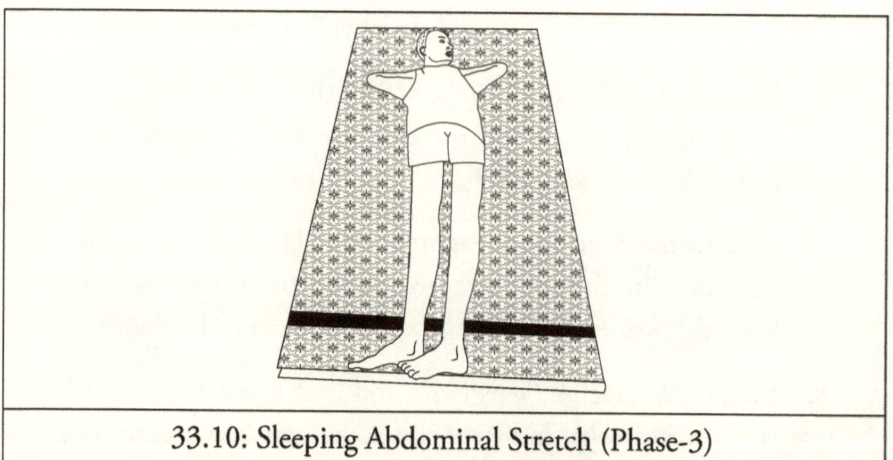

33.10: Sleeping Abdominal Stretch (Phase-3)

10. **Phase – 4:** Now stretch the legs in front. Keeping both legs on ground, make some gap between the big toe and the adjoining finger of left foot. Lift the right leg and place the heel in this gap, i.e., the bottom of right heel will be over the gap between big toe and first finger in left foot. Weight of left foot is being supported by the skin between right toe and adjoining finger. Maintaining the same position, bring the complete assembly of legs to the left side. Allow right toe to touch the ground, left heel resting on ground. Take head to the right side. Now bring the assembly of legs, retaining the right heel on top of left toe arrangement, to the right side and take head to the left side. Try to touch the ground with your nose, and the smallest finger to the ground in opposite directions. Head will always go in directions opposite to the legs. (See 33.11). Complete five to six rounds.

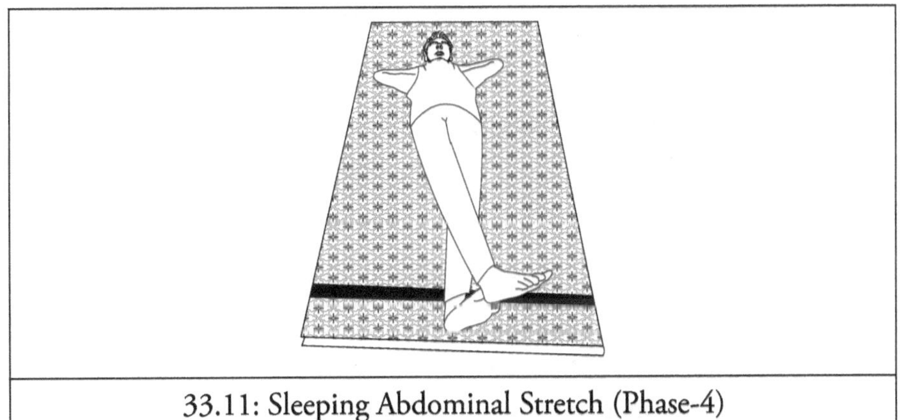

33.11: Sleeping Abdominal Stretch (Phase-4)

11. The Breathing and Focus for Phase-2 to 4 shall remain same as in Phase-1. Bottom portion of head will remain in touch with the ground, smoothly shifting position from left to right and soon.

Exercise Number 33.05: UNIVERSAL SPINAL TWIST POSE

Precautions:

Not to be performed by persons with serious back conditions, back pain, or suffering from any spine related diseases. This exercise rectifies disorders of the hip joint. It should be stopped if the practice is found painful at any stage.

Steps:

1. Lie down flat on the back. (Supine Posture – Base position).

2. Stretch the arms out to the sides at shoulder level with the palms of the hands facing down. Bend the right leg and place the sole of the foot beside the left kneecap. Place the left hand on top of the right knee. This is the starting position.

3. Gently bring the right knee down to the floor on the left side of the body, keeping the leg bent and the foot in contact with the left knee. Turn the head to the right, looking along the straight arm, and gaze at the middle finger of the right hand.

4. The left hand should be on the right knee and the right arm and shoulder should remain in contact with the floor. In the final position, the head should be turned in the opposite direction to the folded knee and the other leg should be completely straight. Hold the position for as long as is comfortable.

5. Return to the starting position, bringing the head and knee to the centre. Stretch the right arm out to the side and straighten the right leg. Repeat on the opposite side. Practise once to each side, gradually extending the holding time. (See 33.12).

33.12: Universal Spinal Twist Posture in Right Side

6. **Breathing:** Inhale in the starting position. Exhale while pushing the knee to the floor and turning the head. Breathe deeply and slowly in the final position. Inhale while centring the body and exhale while straightening the leg.

7. **Focus:** Physical – on the breath or the relaxation of the back.

8. **Sequence:** This asana should be performed after forward and backward bending Asanas or those that are strenuous on the lower back, and after sitting in chairs or in Meditation Asanas for extended periods of time.

Exercise Number 33.06: YOGIC BOAT POSTURE: (NAUKASANA)

Precautions:

Not to be performed by persons with serious back conditions, back pain, or suffering from any spine/nerve related diseases. This asana rectifies disorders of the hip joint. It should be stopped if the practice is painful.

Steps:

1. Lie down flat on the back, i.e., starting posture of Shavasana. (Supine Posture-Base position). Keep hands by the sides, palms down.

2. Keep the eyes open throughout. Breathe in deeply. Hold the breath and then raise the legs, arms, shoulders, head and trunk

off the ground. The shoulders and feet should be not more than 15 cm off the floor. Balance the body on the buttocks and keep the spine straight. The arms should be held at the same level and in line with the toes. Allow your complete body to attain the shape of bottom portion of a boat.

3. The hands should be open with the palms down. Look towards the toes. Remain in the final position and hold the breath. Count to five mentally (or for longer if possible). Breathe out and return to the supine position. Be careful not to injure the back of the head while returning to the floor. Relax the whole body. This is one round. Practise three to five rounds.

4. Relax in Shavasana after each round, gently pushing out the abdomen with inhalation to relax the stomach muscles.

5. **Variation-1:** Repeat Step 1 and 2 and reach the boat posture. Count to five retaining the breath. Now make five to ten swift upwards movements of hands and feet, (just like an infant does when in agitated and demanding mood). Both hands and legs should not be travelling together. When left hand is swiftly going up, right hand should be coming down. Similar should be the state of leg movements. Knees may be bent suitably to achieve smooth, somewhat jerky movements of legs. You may continue the up down movements of hand and legs till fatigued out. Relax in Shavasana till breathing becomes normal again. Chant some relaxation mantra during relaxing to hasten up the relaxing phase.

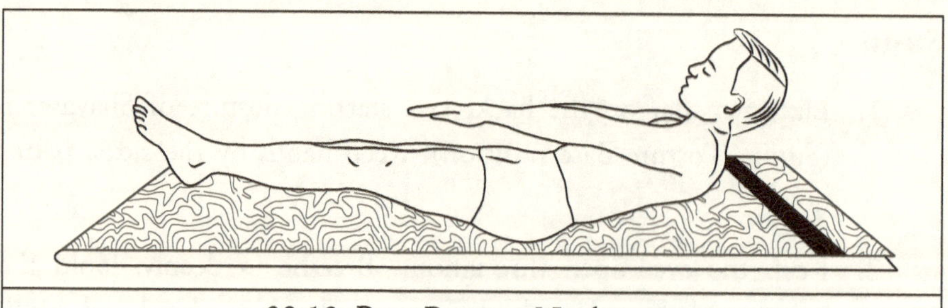

33.13: Boat Posture: Naukasana

6. **Breathing:** Inhale before raising the body. Retain the breath while raising, tensing and lowering the body. Exhale in the base position.

7. **Focus:** Mind: Focussed on the breath, movement, mental counting and tensing of the body (especially the abdominal muscles) in the final position.

8. **Variation-2:** Repeat the same process as above but clench the fists and tense the whole body as much as possible in the raised position. You may also perform the forceful up and down movements of hands and legs in this variation too. The movements of fist shall be akin to boxer's punch. Movements of legs should be like kicking.

Day Thirty-Four: The Subtle Exercises for Upper Body and Cardiac System

Learning and Practice for the Day

Exercise Number 34.01: YOGIC WEIGHTLIFTING

Steps:

1. Sit on the floor, in starting posture, Prarambhiksthithi (Base position) with the legs straight and together (Posture Number S1).

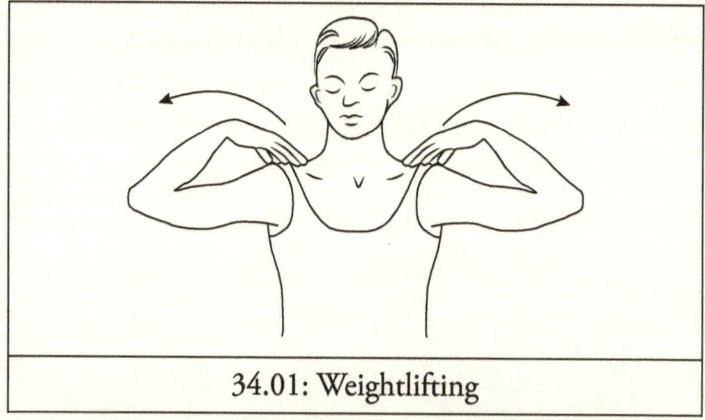

34.01: Weightlifting

2. Keep the eyes open. Open your arms and place them outwards, away from your body at shoulder level, palms facing upwards, parallel to the ground, slightly stretched outwards.

3. Imagine that there are about 10 to 15 Kilograms of weights placed on your arms, close the fist, imagining fist being very heavy due to holding of weights.

4. Now lift both the arms simultaneously and bring the palms over the shoulders. Allow the fingers, joined together forming a circle with all fingers in same plane to touch the shoulder. (See 34.01). Hold for three to five seconds.

5. Bring the arms back to base position. Hold for two to three seconds and then bring down and allow bottom of fist to touch the ground. Lift hands again and take them back on shoulders in one smooth upward circular motion. Again, allow fingers to touch the shoulders. This is one round. Practise five to ten rounds.

6. **Breathing:** Breathe in while taking the arms up and breathe out when arms are coming down.

Exercise Number 34.02: PULLING THE ROPES

Steps:

1. Sit on the floor, in starting posture with the legs straight and together (Posture Number S1). Keep the eyes open. Imagine that there are two ends of a rope hanging in front of the body.

2. You are required to grab the rope-ends and forcefully pull the rope towards you. Breathe in while reaching up with the right hand as though to grasp the rope at a higher point. Keep the elbow straight. Look upwards.

3. While breathing out, slowly pull the right arm down, putting extra power into the arms as though pulling the rope downwards. Let the eyes follow the downward movement of the hand. Repeat with the left hand and arm to complete the first round. Both arms do not move at the same time. Practise five to ten rounds.

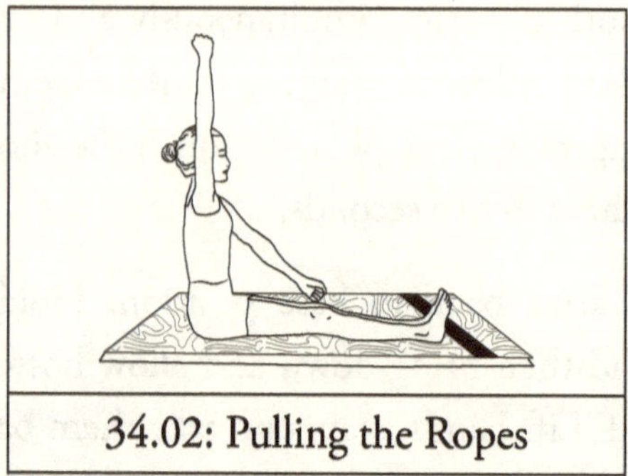

34.02: Pulling the Ropes

4. **Breathing:** Inhale while raising the arm. Exhale while lowering the arm.

5. **Focus:** Mind focussed on the breath, movement and stretch of the upper back and shoulder muscles.

6. **Benefits:** This asana loosens the shoulder joints and stretches the upper back muscles. It firms the breast and develops the muscles of the chest.

Exercise Number 34.03: DYNAMIC SPINAL TWIST

Steps:

1. Sit on the floor with both legs outstretched. Separate the legs as far apart as possible. Do not allow the knees to bend. Stretch the arms sideways at shoulder level. Keeping the arms straight, twist to the left and bring the right hand down towards the left big toe.

2. Stretch the straight left arm behind the back as the trunk twists to the left. Keep both arms in one straight line. Turn the head to the left and gaze at the left outstretched hand. (See 34.03).

3. Twist in the opposite direction and bring the left hand down towards the right big toe. Stretch the straight right arm behind the back. Turn the head to the right and gaze at the right

outstretched hand. This is one round. Practise ten to twenty rounds. Start slowly and then gradually increase the speed.

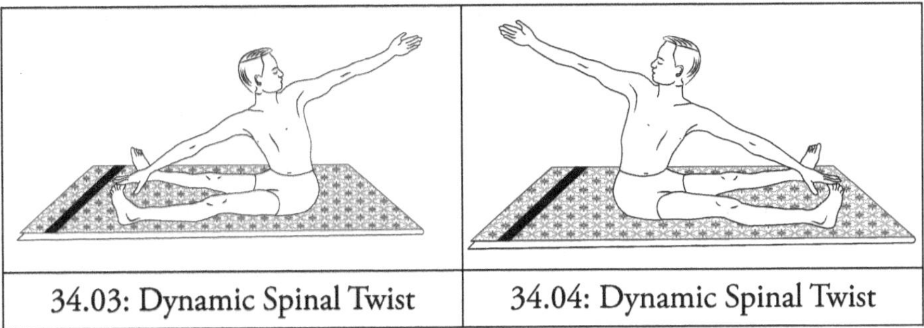

| 34.03: Dynamic Spinal Twist | 34.04: Dynamic Spinal Twist |

4. **Breathing:** To apply pressure in the abdomen: breathe in when twisting and breathe out when returning to the centre. To give maximum flexion of the spine: breathe out when twisting and breathe in when returning to the centre.

5. **Focus:** Mind focussed on the breath, the twisting movement and the effect on the spinal vertebrae and muscles.

Exercise Number 34.04: YOGIC WAY OF ROWING THE BOAT: (NAUKA-VIHAR OR NAUKA-SANCHALANA ASANA)

Steps:

1. This boat rowing exercises may be performed with two variations as described.

2. **Phase – 1:**

Sit with both legs joined together and placed straight in front of the body. Imagine the action of rowing a boat. Clench the hands as though grasping oars, with the palms facing downwards.

Breathe out and bend forward from the waist as far as is comfortable, straightening the arms. Breathing in, lean back as far as possible, drawing the hands back towards the shoulders. This is one round.

The hands should make a complete circular movement in every round, moving up the sides of the legs and trunk. The legs should be kept straight throughout. Do not allow rising of knees; keep them firmly nailed down.

Imagine that your girlfriend or boyfriend is sailing with you in the boat that you are rowing. Make an impressive display of your physical prowess in rowing. Practise five to ten rounds.

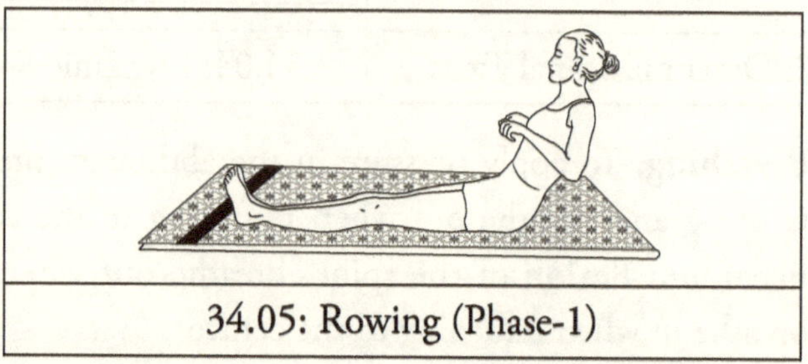

34.05: Rowing (Phase-1)

3. Reverse the direction of the rowing movement as though going in the opposite direction. Practise five to ten times.

4. **Phase – 2:**

    In the same sitting position, spread the legs so that the feet are about one metre apart or as spread out as feasible. The legs should remain straight throughout the practice.

    Repeat the procedure as given in Phase 1. First row over the right leg, then the left leg, and then over the space between the feet.

5. **Breathing:** Inhale while leaning back. Exhale while bending forward.

6. **Focus: Mind:** Focussed on the breath, movement and lower back and pelvic area. Eyes: Preferably closed, if open, focussed on the tips of hands, mentally guiding the hands make as smooth and as powerful a motion as required for steering the boat in a serene, still and beautiful lake.

Exercise Number 34.05: YOGIC WAY OF GRINDING WHEAT (CHAKKI CHALANA ASANA) (Churning the manual mill)

Steps:

1. **Phase – 1:**

   Sit with the legs stretched out in front of the body about one foot apart. Interlock the fingers of both hands and hold the arms out straight in front of the chest. Keep the arms straight and horizontal throughout the practice; do not bend the elbows. Bend forward as far as possible.

   Imagine the action of churning old-style manual grinding mill with an old-fashioned stone grinder. (It used to have two flat circular stones, placed one over another on common axis, the bottom one stationary and top to be rotated manually, wheat passing through the space between wheels, and 'Atta' (flour) used to come out from all sides).

   Swivel to the right so that the hands pass above the right toes and as far to the right as possible. Lean back as far as possible on the backward swing. Try to move the body from the waist. On the forward swing, bring the arms and hands to the left side, over the left toes and then back to the centre position. One rotation is one round. Practise eight to sixteen rounds clockwise and then the same number of rounds anti-clockwise.

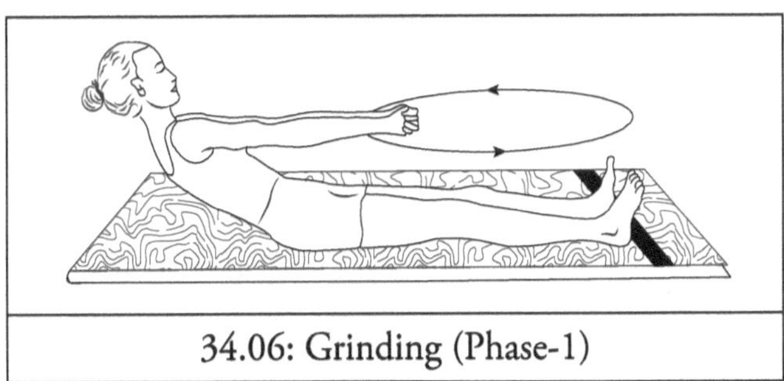

34.06: Grinding (Phase-1)

2. **Phase – 2:**

   In the same sitting position, separate the legs as wide as possible, keeping them straight individually. Make large, circular movements over both feet, again trying to take the hands over the toes on the forward swing and coming as far back as possible on the backward swing. Practise ten times in each direction.

3. **Breathing:** Inhale while leaning back. Exhale while moving forward.

4. **Focus: Mind:** Focussed on the breath, movement and lower back, hips and pelvic area.

5. **Note:** If you find this practise strenuous, appreciate the efforts of your grandmothers/mother, who were routinely grinding the wheat or other grains to feed the family and children, before electricity was invented.

Day Thirty-Five: The Subtle Exercises in Standing Postures

Learning and Practice for the Day

You should, based on your learnings so far, be able to make an accurate prediction, on what I am going to say in introduction to this series. I am still required to perform my duties and discharge my obligations.

The subtle exercises in this series are for those persons, who are always in search of some quick-fix remedies. If you can't spare time and find a place to sit comfortably to perform some simple subtle exercises, and have patience, time and space, only to stand in some open space for a few minutes, this series is especially tailor-made for you.

Here also the stretches are to be performed sequentially. After you obtain mastery over your complete self (body, mind, heart and soul) and the subject of Yoga, you may temper with sequencing, to suit your needs. Till that time follow my advice. My recommended sequencing is, start with loosening up the spine-hip joint, exercise spine, and thereafter travel from toes to head, exercising all major organs one by one.

Depending upon time, patience and your specific needs, you may skip one or two steps in between, but by and large try and follow the sequence. Synchronising breathings with actions, focus of attention, counting, timings, relaxations and all other prerequisites are applicable here too. The general way of breathing (default settings) are:

Inhale: While bending backwards and taking body sideways and while shifting body from front-inclined position to central position.

Retain: While holding the posture.

Exhale: While bending in front and bringing body back from sideways to normal central position.

Relax: In Tadasana, arms loose, breathing through the mouth.

Focus: On the organ primarily involved in exercises, stretches or rotations, and on mentally counting.

35.01: Starting Posture: Prayer/Namaskara Posture

➢ Stand erect in 'Tadasana' with eyes closed, arms hanging loosely downwards, feet together, the body erect, spine straight (if required, perform two to three mild upwards stretches for upper body to keep spine truly vertical) and head held high.

➢ Now fold your hands with the thumbs on the throat-cavity (sternal notch) and the forearms pressed against the chest (Namaskar mudra). Concentrate your mind on the focal point. If feasible, paint a beautiful picture in your mind, place it in front of the focal point, visible to you only with eyes closed.

➢ As soon as you have attained this mental state, relax the pressure of your forearms and palms. Keep the forearms pressed against the chest, till you are unsuccessful in achieving this state of mental concentration.

➢ Retain the posture, breathing normally through nostrils, for one to three minutes. Release and relax! You may also 'Say some prayer' or 'Chant some mantra' or do 'Aum' recitations to strengthen the mental focus, relaxation and meditation.

Spinal Group

35.02: Loosening the Spine-Hip Joint

➤ Stand straight with legs joined together.

➤ Keeping the legs straight, joined together, and hips firmly in position, slowly swing the upper body like pendulum, from above the hips and along with head, sideways, i.e., towards left and right.

➤ Slide your palms along the thighs, such that when upper body is in extreme left position the fingertips of left hand reach up to left knee. Similarly, when body is in extreme right position the fingertips of right palm touch the right knee. (See 35.02).

➤ Repeat the above set three to five times with one more variation. Keep legs about one foot (12 inches) apart and raise both arms at shoulder height.

➤ Keep arms parallel to ground, fingers pointed, arms and palm stretched. Perform swinging actions in left and right, in front and back and twisting actions all as before.

➤ You may keep hands horizontally stationary or involve them in swinging and twisting actions as is found more comfortable.

35.03: Rotating the Upper Body

➤ Stand straight with your legs about one foot apart. Inhale and bring your hands together above the head. Join the palms in 'Namaskar mudra.' Release hands and stand erect.

➤ Exhale and bend forward from the waist keeping the knees straight. Inhale, rotate your upper body to the left, continue inhaling and bend to the back.

➤ Exhale and bend to the right, continue exhaling and bend forward. Inhale and go back, rotate to the right, keep inhaling and rotate to the back.

- Exhale and rotate to the left. Keep exhaling and rotate to the front, get back to initial standing posture.

- This completes one round. Perform three to five rounds.

Note: It is advisable that for practices after this point onwards you take some support. You may stand near a railing, if practising in balcony or place a chair alongside for support. You may support your body with one hand and keep the other hand free. Some practices may however, require you to take support with both hands.

35.04: Spinal Stretches

- Standing erect take support of railing, or chair, with both hands, inhaling deeply, raise and balance your body weight on toes and simultaneously take your head backwards, thus giving your spine a bow like shape.

- Retain the posture and the breath.

- Exhaling smoothly and in circular manner bring the body in front, balance body weight on heels and bring head so that chin is touching the collarbones. The spine has thus again acquired a bow like shape in the opposite direction.

- Retain the posture and the breath.

- Release the posture and inhaling deeply return to the normal posture. This was one round. Perform two to five rounds.

35.05: Swinging Poses

- Stand straight and erect with your legs apart. Raise the arms over the head, keeping the elbows straight and palms joined together.

- Bend forward and swing the trunk down from the hips.

- Allow the arms and head to swing through the legs.

- Be relaxed, tension-free like a soft puppet.

➢ Return smoothly to the upright position with the arms raised.

➢ Inhale deeply and forcefully through the nose while raising the arms up and exhale forcefully while swinging downwards. Repeat five to ten times.

Leg Group

35.06: Toe Bending, Ankle Bending and Rotation Exercises

➢ Standing erect take support of railing, or chair, with one hand, keeping other hand free. Balance your body weight on left leg and take your right leg slightly in front, about 12 inches away and 1 to 2 inches above ground.

➢ Recollect your learning of Exercise Number 27.01 (Toe bending exercise). Focus attention on right toes. Stretch and release the toes to cause five to twelve to-and-fro movements. Count five to twelve movements.

➢ Similarly recollecting and correlating the learnings of Exercise Number 27.02 (Ankle bending exercise) make five to twelve to-and-fro movements of right foot around the ankle.

➢ Utilising the skills acquired from Exercise Number 27.03 (Ankle rotation exercise) perform five to twelve clockwise and anti-clockwise rotations of right foot, keeping knee and heel rigidly fixed.

➢ Release the posture and relax!

➢ Balancing the body weight on right leg, repeat the above set with left leg and left foot.

35.07: Knee Bending and Rotation Exercise

➢ Retain the posture and the breath. Release the posture and relax. This was one round. You may repeat for five to twelve rounds.

➤ If you can comfortably balance your body weight on one leg, utilise both hands for exercise; else use one hand for support and one for exercise. Choice is yours.

➤ Balancing weight on left leg, place both or one palm below right thigh near the knee joint, making effort to support the thigh, such that it gets raised up and placed parallel to ground, and right leg below knee remains vertical to the ground.

➤ Rotate clockwise the leg below knee around the knee joint for five to twelve rotations. Repeat five to twelve rotations in anti-clockwise directions. This is like Exercise Number 28.04, i.e., knee rotation exercise.

➤ Release the posture and relax.

➤ Repeat the same set for left leg, maintaining body weight on right leg.

35.08: Hip Rotations

➤ Standing erect take support of railing, or chair, with both hands or one hand, as is more comfortable. Balance your body weight on left leg, tilting the body slightly towards left. Take your right leg slightly in front, about 12 inches away and 1 to 2 inches above ground.

➤ From this position smoothly rotate the complete right leg around the hip junction socket, in rotational movements to resemble as if the right big toe or right heel is drawing up a circle on the ground. Keep spine straight and vertical. Do not allow body to swing leftwards or rightwards. Utilise your learning from Exercise Number 28.06 for this exercise.

➤ Repeat for five to ten rotations in clockwise and five to ten rotations in anti-clockwise directions.

➤ Repeat the same set for left leg.

I think it shall be an exercise in futility, if I tell you that you may similarly perform all the subtle exercises for the hands, eyes, shoulder rotations and wrist rotations, etc. based on your previous learnings. I am therefore illustrating only a few more of the exercises below. Utilise your knowledge of exercising all important organs from head to toe and subtle exercises of sitting posture series (Day-Twenty-seven to Day Thirty-one) to fill up the gaps.

35.09: Shoulder Rotations

➢ Stand straight with your legs joined together.

➢ Place your hands on the shoulders, fingers joined together forming a small circle, fingers pointing downwards placed on shoulder-arm joint.

➢ Breathe normally.

➢ Start rotating your arms in big circles towards the backside first and then in front (Right-anti-clockwise, left-clockwise). Allow your elbows to kiss each other when crossing your vision line. Use skin of arms to give gentle massage to your cheeks. Repeat five circles.

➢ Repeat rotation towards the front (Right-clockwise, left-anti-clockwise) for five circles.

➢ Release the hands and get back to initial standing pose and relax.

35.10: Wrists Rotations

➢ Stand straight erect with your legs joined together.

➢ Bring your hands in front on the shoulder level.

➢ Start rotating your both wrists with closed fist.

➢ Rotate five circles to the outer side (Right-clockwise, left-anti-clockwise), then five circles in the opposite direction.

➤ Place the wrists, fists closed over the ears, rotate around the ears, five circles to the outer side (Right-clockwise, left-anti-clockwise), then five circles in the opposite direction.

➤ Release the hands and get back to initial standing pose. Relax.

35.11: Neck Movements and Rotations

➤ Stand straight erect with your legs apart.

➤ Bring your hands on the waist, place hands firmly on the hips to ensure steady state of body portion below hips.

➤ Tilt the neck to the right, allow right earlobe to kiss the shoulder-arm joint, take it back to central position and then towards the left in smooth, jerk-free movements. Allow left earlobe to kiss the left shoulder. Repeat five to ten times.

➤ Similarly perform backwards and front movements of neck five to ten times. Maintain breath synchronisation.

➤ Now bend the neck forward and start rotating to the left, to the back, to the right and front (Anti-clockwise). Repeat five to ten times.

➤ Now rotate back to the right, back, left and front (Clockwise) five to ten times.

➤ Straighten the neck and release the hands, come back to the initial standing pose.

Many of the exercises of Standing Posture Series and Sitting Posture Series (Day Twenty-seven to Day Thirty-one) may also be performed sitting comfortably on a chair with some modifications and compromises. The accrued benefits may be inferior to those of actual practice and may take somewhat longer time to show results.

Day Thirty-Six: The Subtle Exercises for Eyes

Learning and Practice for the Day

The technology-obsessed lifestyle has placed lots of screens in front of our eyes. They come in all sizes, shapes, colours, textures, brightness and contrast levels. Each brings its own set of stresses and strains for our eyes. Long periods of reading and watching smaller or larger screens do not cause as much damage as bad posture and stressed conditions of mind and eyes, during such activities, does.

In general, the factors responsible for poor eyesight are improper illumination, prolonged focus on electronic screens, sitting/lying in poor postures with un-relaxed eyes and mind, dietary habits, mental/emotional stresses, and ageing.

One cannot cure major eye disorders, such as Glaucoma, Trachoma, Cataract, Conjunctivitis, etc. with Yoga. However, the Yogic way of life, some routine precautions, good habits and some minor exercises, shall ensure good vision, good eyesight and longevity of eyes. The set of good habits includes:

- Ensure proper, glare-free, uniform illumination, with Lux (SI unit of measurements of light intensity) levels commensurate with the activity, while reading, watching screens and performing other activities requiring focus of eyes. Adopt good dietary habits; you know what they are.

- Splashing cold water (tap water at room temperature) onto the eyes in the early morning and a few times during the day. Take a little water into the palms over a wash basin and splash it over the eyelids.

- Walk with bare feet on the grass, sand or bare earth early in the morning, when the dew is still fresh.

- Relax your eyes by performing the simple exercise of keeping feet about one foot apart, shifting the weight of body onto one side raising the opposite heel off the ground, swinging your body like inverted pendulum back and forth while simultaneously gazing at a fixed point at some distance (keep eyes pivoted and focussed on a point) for a few minutes.

- Saying 'Good Morning' to the rising sun, gazing at it during the first 15 degrees of its trajectory for a few minutes, closing the eyes and focussing on the after image formed in mind/eyes is also a good relaxing exercise for eyes. Even a simple sun bath while facing the rising sun is good. Do this only very early in the morning, when the sun is rising or in the evening, when the sun is setting.

- If using spectacles, take them off, when not required.

Yoga also contains some great exercises having profound, therapeutic effects on eyes. Some of these are described here:

Important Notes

1. Before beginning these subtle exercises beneficial for eyes, splash cold water onto the eyes for at least ten times.

2. All exercises are recommended to be performed in sequential manner, i.e., one after another, in the same order as described. For best results, daily practice is recommended. If time is a constraint,

include this set of exercises in weekend day's package. Patience and perseverance are required for results.

Precautions for Complete Set

Persons suffering from major eyes disorders or diseases, e.g., Glaucoma, Trachoma, Cataract, Iritis, Keratitis, Conjunctivitis, retinal artery or vein thrombosis must consult an eye specialist before practice.

36.01: First Exercise: Palming the Eye Sockets

Sit quietly and close the eyes. Rub the palms of the hands together vigorously until they become red hot. You may also alternatively heat up your hands by vigorous clapping (Recollect: Learning from Package Number 1 of Chapter-Two Day-Twenty-one, 'Packaged Stress Busters'). Place the heated up/red palms gently over the eyelids, without any undue pressure. Breathe normally.

Feel the warmth and energy being transmitted from the hands into the eyes and the eye muscles relaxing. The eyes are being bathed in a soothing darkness. Remain in this position until the heat from the hands has been fully absorbed by the eyes. Then lower the hands, keeping the eyes closed.

Again, rub the palms together/clap until they become hot and place them over the closed eyes. Make sure the bottom portion of palms and not the fingers cover the eyes. The eye cavities should be completely and gently filled up by the skin in the bottom portion of palm. Keep on adjusting the relative positioning of palms to obtain good contact area between the skin of the palms and the eyelids. Repeat this procedure at least three times. You may do up to ten repetitions.

Palming relaxes and revitalises the eye muscles, and stimulates the circulation of the aqueous humour, the liquid that runs between the cornea and the lens of the eye, aiding the correction of defective vision.

Important Note: The benefits get enhanced when the exercise is performed in front of the rising or setting sun. Focus your mind on the warmth of the sun and its light on the closed lids. Never look directly at the sun except for a few initial moments, when it is just rising or when it is about to set. (Trajectory angle < 15 degrees)

36.02: Second Exercise: Blinking the Eyes

Sit with the eyes open. Blink the eyes ten times quickly. Close the eyes and relax for twenty seconds. Repeat the blinking ten times quickly and then again close the eyes and relax. This is one round. Repeat for five rounds.

36.03: Third Exercise: Viewing Sideways

Assume a sitting posture with the legs straight in front of the body, joined together. Raise the arms to the sides at shoulder level, keeping them straight and point the thumbs upwards.

The thumbs should be just in the peripheral vision when the head is facing forward. If they are not clearly visible, bring them slightly forward until they come into view. Don't move the head. Head should remain stationary, in central position throughout the practise. Look at a fixed point directly in front and on a level with the eyes.

Fix the position of the head in this neutral position. Then, without moving the head sideways, focus the eyes on the followings, one after the other: (a) left thumb (b) space between the eyebrows (the focal point) (c) right thumb (d) space between the eyebrows (e) left thumb. Inhale in the neutral position.

Exhale while looking to the sides. Inhale and come to the centre. This is one round. Repeat this cycle for ten to twenty rounds. Keep the head and spine straight throughout. Finally, close and rest the eyes. Palming may be performed several times. If the arms become tired they may be supported on set of pillows, cushions or two stools.

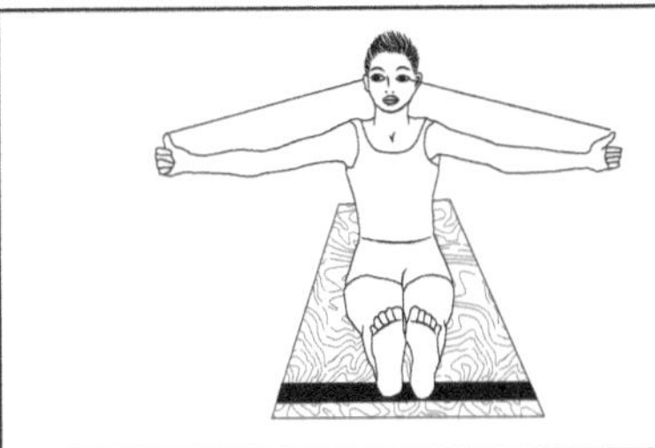

36.01: Third Exercise:
Viewing Sideways

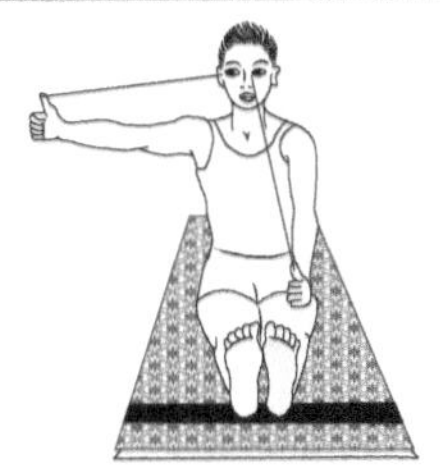

36.02: Fourth Eexercise:
Viewing Sideways and in Front

36.04: Fourth Exercise: Viewing Sideways and In Front

Maintain or assume the same body posture as in third exercise. Place the left thumb on the left knee, so that it points upward. Hold the right thumb to the right of the body so that it points upward.

Note that both hands are placed perpendicular to each other. Head remaining stationary in centre, focus the eyes on the left thumb, then on the right thumb and then return to the left thumb. Inhale in the neutral position.

Exhale while looking down. Inhale while looking up. This is one round. Repeat this process for fifteen to twenty rounds. Then rest and close the eyes. Repeat the same procedure on the left side of the body. Keep the head and spine straight throughout the exercise. Finally, close and rest the eyes. Palming may be performed several times.

36.05: Fifth Exercise: Rotational Viewing

Maintain or assume the same body posture, as it was in fourth exercise. Place the left hand on the left knee. Hold the right fist above the right leg with the right thumb pointing in upward direction and the elbow straight.

Focus eyes on right thumb. Make a large circular movement with the right arm to the left, then upward, curving to the right, and finally returning to the starting position. Try to make as smooth and as large a circle, as feasible. Keep the eyes focussed on the thumb, with head remaining in fixed central position.

Inhale while completing the upper arc of the circle. Exhale while completing the lower arc. The breath should be smooth and synchronised with the forming of the perfect circles. Perform these circular motions five times clockwise and then five times anti-clockwise.

Repeat with the left thumb. Keep the head and spine straight throughout. Finally, close and rest the eyes. Palming may be performed several times.

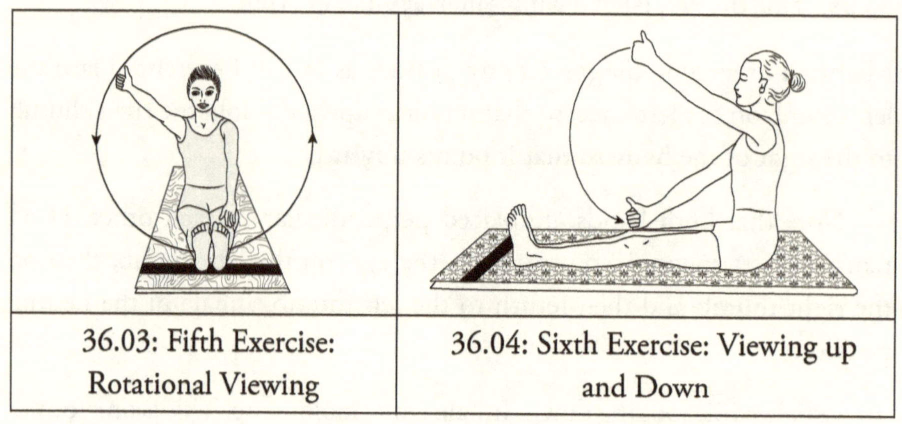

36.03: Fifth Exercise: Rotational Viewing	36.04: Sixth Exercise: Viewing up and Down

36.06: Sixth Exercise: Viewing Up and Down

Maintain or assume the same posture as in fifth exercise. Place both fists on the knees with both thumbs pointing upward. Remember to keep the head and spine straight throughout the exercise and breathing synchronised.

Keeping the arms straight, slowly raise the right thumb, while following the motion of the thumb with the eyes. When the thumb is raised to the maximum, slowly return to the starting position, all the time keeping the eyes focussed on the thumb without moving the head.

Inhale while raising the eyes. Exhale while lowering the eyes. Practise the same movement with the left thumb. Repeat five times with each thumb. Finally, close and rest the eyes. Palming may be performed several times.

36.07: Seventh Exercise: Gazing at Nose Tip

Sit comfortably with the legs straight in front or in any cross-legged pose. Hold the right arm straight directly in front of the nose. Make a fist with the right hand, keeping the thumb pointing upward. Focus both eyes on the tip of the thumb.

Bend the arm and slowly bring the thumb to the nose tip, keeping the eyes focussed on the tip of the thumb. Remain for a few seconds with the thumb held at the nose tip and the eyes focussed there.

Slowly straighten the arm, continuing to gaze at the thumb tip. Breathe in as the thumb is drawn towards the nose. Retain the breath inside while holding the thumb at the nose tip. Breathe out as the arm is straightened. This is one round. Repeat five rounds.

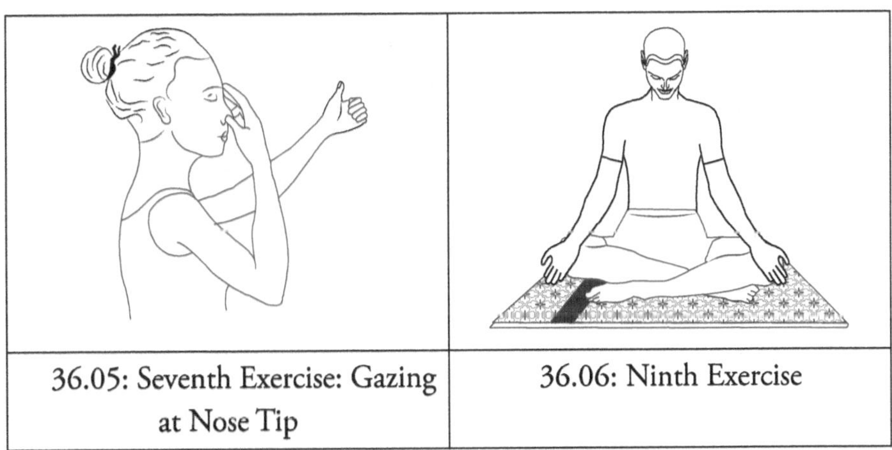

36.05: Seventh Exercise: Gazing at Nose Tip	36.06: Ninth Exercise

36.08: Eighth Exercise: Near and Distant Viewing

Stand or sit at an open window, preferably with a clear view of the horizon, with the arms by the sides. Focus the eyes on the nose tip, for five seconds. Then, focus on an imaginary distant object on the horizon for five seconds. Inhale during near viewing. Exhale during distant viewing. Repeat this process ten to twenty times. Close the eyes and relax. Palming may be performed at this time.

36.09: Ninth Exercise: Viewing Up, In Centre and Down

Stand or sit at an open window, with a clear view of the horizon. If practising indoors without a window facing a clear horizon, stand facing a wall.

Now consciously and mentally mark three imaginary points, either in the horizon or on front wall as follows: (a) First point; vertically up on horizon/wall as high as your eyes may reach, on the wall, this point may be at wall-ceiling joint) (b) Second; in centre, a point you can see with head in normal position and (c) Third; vertically down as low as your eyes may reach. Focus the eyes on the central point (Second point).

Without causing any movement of head and neck, take eyes up and focus on first point. Keep mind and vision focussed on this point for a few seconds. Now bring eyes down and focus on second point, maintaining focus for a few seconds.

Again, bring the eyes down and focus on third point. Take eyes up to the first point, resting for a few seconds on central (Second) point. Inhale when vision is going up, exhale when coming down, retain when focussing. This is one round. Repeat this process for ten to twenty rounds. Close the eyes and relax. Palming may be performed at this time

After completing this series of practices lie in Shavasana for a few minutes.

The proof of the pudding is in the eating. To test the efficacy and effectiveness of this series of exercises, you may conduct a simple experiment. Get your eyes tested by an eye specialist. You know the way they make you read those very small fonts. So, better print an A4 size sheet with font size varying from twenty at top to below eight at bottom. Try to read this sheet from top to bottom and preserve it. Diligently practise this series of Asanas for one month. Now take out that sheet and try reading again from top to bottom. You should be able to see the difference yourself, without paying the fee to the eye specialist.

Day Thirty-Seven: Make Your Own Package of Subtle Exercises

Learning of the Day

Now that you have been reading, learning, assimilating and partly practising Yoga for more than forty days, do not look at the number of days in the heading part of the Chapter and sneer at me. I know you initially took a few extra days and have also skipped learning and practising for some days in between. So, no harm in my assumptions. Anyways, it is time for some revisions, summarisations and recapitulations of your learnings so far.

You have learnt meditation, the most complex Art and Science of Yogic practices. You learnt to control, tame, domesticate and tie on a tight leash your mind, and to make it faithfully obey your commands. The tiger amongst all the organs of your body, is now at your disposal. The aimless wanderer now asks your permission before proceeding on those useless voyages and transgressing into oblivions.

You have learnt to channelize the energy of your mind and the powers of your brain. You can attain focus of mind, the way you want it. Your senses follow your dictates. And you can streamline these energies to give you peace, health, happiness, creativity, imagination, powers of observation and overall wellbeing. Well, if you have still not acquired these proficiencies, it is time to take a break, go back and restart your learning process from Chapter-One, Day-One onwards after some time.

Please understand that there is no point in aimlessly and uselessly pretending to perform Yoga Asanas, with a half-baked skill set, without your mind and heart being engrossed and completely involved in the exercises. The best that you may expect from such exercises is what you could otherwise get by spending that much time in the Gymnasium. The worst is too dangerous to mention here. If proper precautions are not followed, you may even cause injury to yourself.

You are also expected, by now, to master the Art and Science of Pranayama. The power to regulate and channelize your breath, 'the prana.' The ability to utilise the energies associated with your respiratory systems, for your wellbeing. The ability to synchronise your breathings with actions. I will reiterate, even at the cost of being repetitive, do not proceed to Yoga Asanas of Chapter-Five without acquiring a neat, clean, well-polished and shining skill set.

This was the most important Chapter, most important part, of what I intended to teach and the most important for your learning process also. In this Chapter, you have learnt the subtle exercises, the minor exercises, and 'Yogabhyas' (Yogic practices) not requiring much physical efforts.

You have also learnt, as to how to exercise each body part and each internal organ of your body. I have deliberately refrained from mentioning the benefits of each exercise. If you are blessed with good powers of observation, you may conveniently make out the benefits of each exercise, quite accurately. You should by now be familiar with taking good care of your body, from head to toe, from toe to head and from body to soul.

If you have acquired the three skills narrated above, the major portion, say about 90%, of your learning is complete. You may, if you want, skip Chapter-Five and start your daily practice with this skill set. All that is required is to prepare a package of practices, for performing daily, based on your needs and the available time.

Hey! But what about Asanas? The ones that we have seen the people learning or practising Yoga, performing. Aren't we supposed to learn those difficult postures, 'Shirshasana' (Head down standing posture, balancing body weight on skull) or 'Halasana,' 'Eka-Pada-Sarvangasana,'

'Urdhva-Padmasana-in-Sarvangasana' etc. etc.? Aren't they important? Yes! They are important too.

But, their importance lies in advanced practices. They are important for advanced practitioners. They also carry great significance in curative parts of Yoga. They are important for 'sadhaks,' i.e., those in search of some spiritual enlightenment and connections, cosmic energies and suffering with insatiable hungers towards quest of the 'truth,' absolute knowledge and answers to most complex, unanswered questions of life and universe, its origin and purpose etc. etc.

For commoners like you and I, the basics and the spirit of Yoga are more important than advanced asana. A very few of the Asanas are covered in Chapter-Five. Here also I shall be including the easier ones only. The 'Soul' of Yoga is already covered up till this Chapter. Once you have mastered the soul, you can keep on adding the flesh, blood and bones from advanced learnings to this soul, to create your body of Yoga. You may now conveniently start some real, serious and confident practice.

I have already hinted, more than once so far, that you need to build up your own package of routine practices, based on your needs, your priorities and your availability of time that can be spared. If you have understood this concept well, nothing more is required, go ahead build your package for daily practising. Start practising, keep on learning, keep on adding new practices from new learnings, keep on observing and experimenting, keep on modifying based on observations and experimentation and finally keep on re-assessing, re-evaluating your needs and priorities and thus keep on changing the package. I am now going to faint from fatigue of counting my 'keep on.'

If you haven't mastered the concepts yet, you deserve and therefore need to go through the painful process of understanding my following explanations and elaborations.

The first issue that needs to be well understood is that the concepts of 'spare-able-time' and 'time constraints' are non-existent, imaginary and hypothetical perceptions of mind. These are mental-blocks only. These are part of the classical approach of your brain to befool you. If you sincerely believe that your time is so precious, that you cannot afford to waste, 45×365 minutes of it, on your wellbeing, fools' paradise is your abode. Imagine what will happen if you fall sick and are hospitalised. Will heaven fall on earth? Will all hell break loose? Will Sun, Moon, Air, Water and everything else forget their duties and responsibilities? Believe me! Nothing of this sort will happen. It will affect only your wallet, your bank balance, your body, your life-balance and may be, your immediate family and the near and dear ones. No one else will even come to know, when and why you fell sick, when you were hospitalised, when discharged and how much was the bill for, except may be your medical-insurance-provider. And he cares a damn about you. He will only curse you for falling sick. So, leave those lame excuses aside, and get on to the real business of taking really good care of yourself.

Your needs and priorities are dependent upon lots of factors, the more important ones, being your age, family profile and your educational/ professional profiles. Let's try and understand these typical needs and priorities one by one.

If you are at the elementary education stage (below class 10th, age between eight and fifteen years) your priorities are more likely to be, getting up from the bed in time each day early morning, without getting a mouthful from mother/father, going through the elaborate, cumbersome process of daily grind of routines, catching the transport just-in-time to reach school, making those extra efforts to not fall asleep during classes, pass with good marks/grades those stressful weekly or monthly exams and most important to avoid, at all costs the situations to feel small or inferior in front of that Chemistry/English teacher. It is not that you have some crush on him/her, but he/she is so cute, so handsome/beautiful. It doesn't feel good. No belittling in front of him/her please!

You are in a different and much more complex situation, if you have crossed the elementary education stage (age group fifteen to twenty-five).

There are those Parental and Societal pressures of choosing the right career, the right profession, getting into the right coaching, the right college or right university. And then there are those urges, some of body, some of passions, some of creativities and some of unknown/unexplained varieties. All adding to the burden of stresses. And to add salt to injuries, there are those pains of so-and-so getting ahead of you, taking along the best girl/guy of the class, getting better grades and qualifying those tough competitive examinations. Net result is stresses beyond comprehension.

The space of one full book is insufficient to describe the intricacies of the family and work-related stresses. If you may somehow categorise and define one-hundred types of stresses, you may also conveniently come across someone claiming to be suffering from one-hundred-and-ten types of stresses.

Similarly, if you are suffering from the pains or enjoying the fun of your recent superannuation from work-life, your priorities of making smooth changeovers are likely to be different. In old age the knee pains and the back pains are the biggest issues of life, everything else is peanuts.

The point that I am trying to make here is that, with age the priorities of life keep on changing. Correspondingly the needs that we expect Yoga to fulfil, also keep on changing. Similar variations in needs and priorities are expected depending upon the educational and professional profiles, family-profiles, the financial status and many other parameters of an individual. Just as one medicine cannot be prescribed for all ailments, one universally applicable package of Yogic practices cannot be designed. One must access his needs realistically and design a package for himself.

Hey! How about the tiny toddlers, the infant ones? Why didn't you consider them? Oh! Sorry! I became greedy. I know none of them is expected to be reading this book. So, took the liberty of ignoring them. And they as such are in the most beautiful phase of their life. No stress! No hassles! I cannot teach them anything. They need no learning also. We need to learn from them, emulate their ways and actions in our life and find time once in a while to relive our childhood days.

As Yoga enthusiast my advice to parents is, if you are convinced about the utility of Yoga, initiate your kids also into it, as early as possible. In young age bones are flexible and joints are supple. It is easier for them. They will pick up even the seemingly complex Asanas very fast. They may turn out to be role models for you. Teach them a posture, observe them perfecting it fast, and then you chase their progress, copy them and perfect your postures.

Let me come back to the topic of assisting and guiding you in deciding your package of practices, if you are still stuck with it. I am giving suggestive break-up for a minimalistic sixty minutes package. One may proportionately adjust for thirty to 100-minute duration package. If time available is below thirty minutes, just concentrate on Meditation and Pranayama. More than hundred minutes of daily practice for a commoner is not recommended.

Table for the Day

Age Profile (Years)	Recommended time-spread in daily package of practices. (Minutes)			
	Meditation	Pranayama	Sukshma-Vyayama	Relaxation and rest
10–15	15	20	20	05
15–25	20	20	10	10
25–60	10	20	20	10
60 Plus	05–10	15–20	15–20	15

Now the only query that remains unanswered is how to pick and choose some subtle exercises from the large set of exercises of this Chapter for your working days and weekend day's package. Till the time you acquire the qualifications of a 'Yoga-Sadhak,' 'Yoga Teacher,' 'Yoga Guru' or a 'Yoga-Acharya' do not even think of attempting all the exercises every day.

The one series of exercises involving one specific organ, say eyes, spinal flexibility or specific joints may be included in your weekend package depending upon your specific needs. Now the other important criterion you need to satisfy is that your package must include something for everyone, i.e., cover yourself from head to toe or toe to head.

At forty plus age, your package must pay specific attention to the spine and lower spinal joints. At sixty plus age the flexibility, suppleness, greasing and lubrication of knee joints, lower back joints and neck joints along with dentures and eyes should be focal point of practices.

My last piece of advice in this Chapter is, do not take these subtle exercises lightly. It is advised to follow a ten-ten-ten days of Pretend – Attempt – Practise learning schedule.

For the first ten days just pretend that you are performing these subtle exercises. Just try and imitate the posture, without making any extra efforts to attain perfection in postures. For the next ten days make some real attempts to learn the intricacies of perfections in posture and only after twenty days of pretending and learning, make some real attempts at perfection in performances. This way you shall reach a good level of proficiency in one-month duration.

Chapter-Five

The Yoga Asana

Chapter–Five

Day Thirty-Eight: The Yoga Asana in Standing Posture: Part – I

Learning and Practice for the Day

Is there any need to define Yoga Asana? These are the most visible, most advertised, prominent and profound parts of Yoga. We will begin our learning of this power-packed package by saluting the Sun, the omnipotent source of freely available energies for all human, animal and plant life, on this planet Earth.

38.01: The Sun Salutation Postures: Surya-Namaskara

The Sun salutation posture is not one isolated Asana; it is a package of twelve postures. It is, in fact a complete package of exercises involving all major organs. If all that you can manage is just a ten to fifteen minutes time-slot from your busy schedule, just perform two to three complete rounds of this Asana. You will get at least 50% of the benefits of an otherwise one-hour long bouquet of other formats of physical exercises. It is such a powerful package.

Do understand and master each stage carefully. It is an effective way of loosening up, stretching, massaging and toning up all the joints, muscles and internal organs of the body. It is invariably recommended with mantra recitations and meditation techniques. I am however, covering the physical aspects of postures only, leaving the spiritual parts aside. Do look up in advanced books, if interested in spiritually-enriched versions.

The ideal time to practise is at sunrise. It is the ideal way of saying 'Good Morning' to the Sun, the source of solar energy.

Precautions

Immediately stop the practice, if a feverish condition, acute inflammation, boils or rashes occur. These conditions may appear due to extreme levels of toxins in your body. Get yourself detoxed properly and return to the practice.

Persons suffering from high blood pressure, coronary artery diseases, poor heart conditions (those who have had a stroke) should not attempt this. Avoid in cases of hernia and intestinal tuberculosis.

People with back conditions must consult a Medical/Yoga expert. Girls should not practise during onset of menstruation, during pregnancy, and up to fifty days after child-birth.

Steps:

Position 1:

Before starting the practice, stand comfortably with feet together or slightly apart. Fold your hands in 'Namaskar Mudra' and spend a few seconds in meditation. You should have no issues in saying some prayers in praise of the selfless energy dispenser. This pose is prayer pose called 'PRANAMASANA' in Hindi.

Now, lower the arms and stand loose. Arms should be hanging loosely by the side of the body. Close your eyes gently and start mentally focussing on your body, traversing from head to toe and vice-versa, relaxing all organs.

Your body may tend to sway from side to side or backwards-forwards. Try to stabilize the body, minimizing the oscillations. The body weight should be equally balanced on both feet (two points). Keep breathing normally.

First take the mental focus inside the body, mentally observing all internal organs from top to bottom and relaxing them. Then retaining the mental focus inside the body, allow the focus to travel upwards from bottom to top.

Thereafter, allow the mind and all senses to focus on soles of feet in contact with ground. Relax the complete body releasing all tensions. Allow the focus to traverse over the complete body externally from bottom to top and top to bottom, releasing tensions in all body parts and relaxing the parts.

Finally, take the focus of mind on the focal point of all senses. Mentally visualise and paint a picture of the beautiful, brilliant, red-hot, fresh, energetic rising sun, and establish this picture at focal point. Each movement, each transition from this position to all subsequent positions, must be with smooth synchronised movements, as if dancing to please that one person, who matters the most to you.

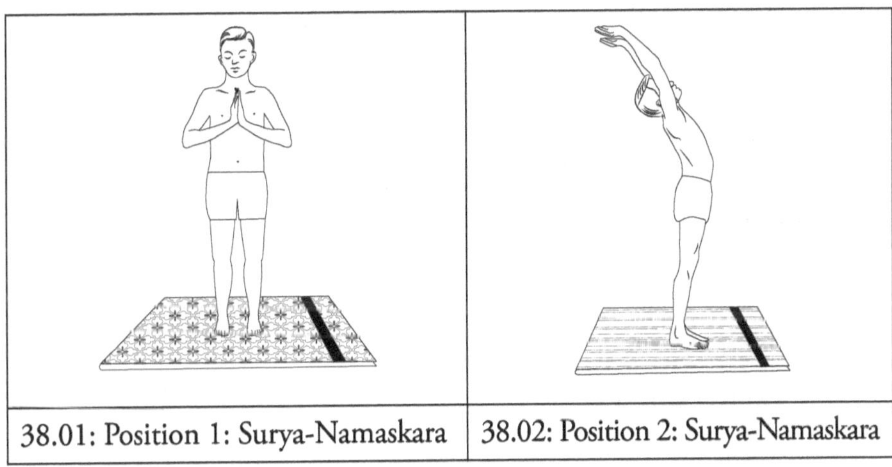

| 38.01: Position 1: Surya-Namaskara | 38.02: Position 2: Surya-Namaskara |

Position 2:

Raise and stretch both arms above the head. Keep the arms separated, at shoulder width apart. Inhaling deeply bend the head, arms and upper trunk backwards. Take your hands and back as much backwards as feasible, keeping the flexibility of lower back joints in view and keeping the legs straight.

Keep the mind focussed on the stretch of the abdomen and expansion of the lungs. Body weight is supported by the two feet. The heels are carrying the extra burden for providing balance. This raised armed pose is called 'HASTA UTTAN ASANA.'

Position 3:

(Note: If suffering from back conditions, do not bend forward fully. Bend from the hips keeping the spine straight, until the back forms close to ninety-degree angle with the legs. Better still, bend only as far as comfortable.)

Now from position 2, exhaling forcefully, bend forward, smoothly, until the fingers or palms of the hands touch the floor on either side of the feet. Try to touch the knees with forehead. If touching knees is not feasible bring forehead as close to knees as feasible.

Do not overstrain. Knees should be straight. Try to contract the abdomen in the final position to expel the maximum amount of air from the lungs. Keep mind focussed on the pelvic region, feeling the compression. Weight of body is being transferred smoothly through legs and feet. Hands are providing supports only for maintaining balance. This hand to foot pose is called 'PADAHASTASANA.'

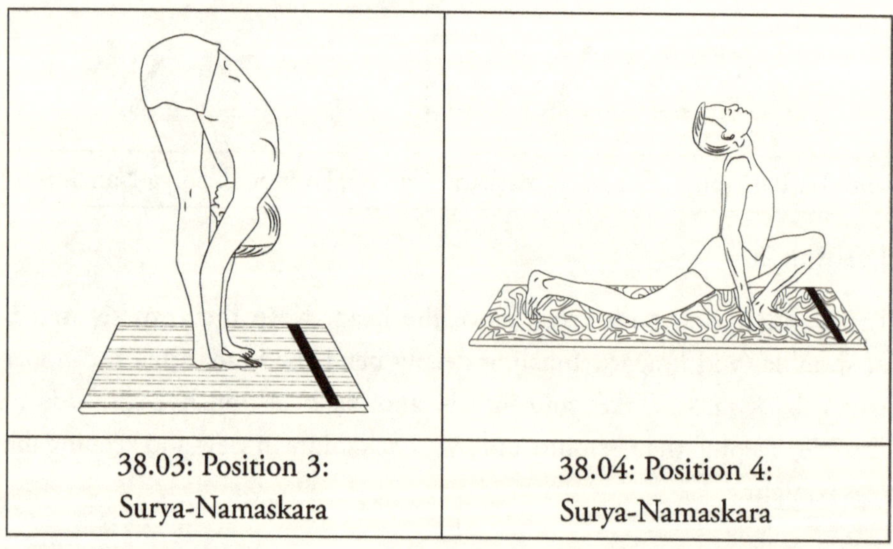

38.03: Position 3: Surya-Namaskara	38.04: Position 4: Surya-Namaskara

Position 4:

From position 3, place the palms of the hands flat on the floor besides the feet. Inhale deeply and stretch the right leg back as far as possible. Simultaneously, bend the left knee, keeping the left foot on the floor in the same position.

Keep the arms straight. In the final position, the weight of the body should be uniformly supported by both hands, the left foot, the right knee and toes of the right foot (i.e., load transferring to ground via five points).

The head should be tilted backwards; keep the back arched and focus of mind on the focal point. Maintain focus of mind on the stretch from the thigh to the chest and/or on the focal point.

In final pose only, beginners should keep the palms of the hands on the floor. Later, as you become advanced practitioners, the body weight should be supported on fingertips, instead of palms. This equestrian like pose is named 'ASHWA SANCHALANASANA.'

Position 5:

Migrating from position 4, exhale deeply and take the left foot back beside the right foot. At the same time, raise the buttocks and lower the head between the arms, so that the back and hands form one line and legs form second line of the triangular shape of the body.

The legs and arms should be straight in the final position. Breathe normally as required. Do not allow bending of arms at elbows. Try to keep heels on the floor in final pose and bring the head towards the knees.

Do not over strain. The body weight should be uniformly transferred to ground through hands and heels of feet (four points). Keep the mind focussed on relaxing the hips or on the throat region (under compression). This mountain resembling posture is called 'PARVATASANA.'

38.05: Position 5: Surya-Namaskara	38.06: Position 6: Surya-Namaskara

Position 6:

This position needs deeper understandings. So, pay attention! Transiting from position 5 exhale, you must retain the breath outside in this final pose. After exhaling, lower the knees, chest and chins slowly on to the floor.

Keep the hips slightly upwards, pointing towards the sky. In the final position only the toes, knees, chest, hands and chin touch the floor. The knees, chest and chin should touch the floor simultaneously and smoothly. If some difficulties are faced, first lower the knees, then the chest, and finally the chin.

The buttocks, hips and abdomen should be raised. Belly flesh should not touch the ground. There should be enough space, below the pelvic region, for air to pass through. Retain the breath during this pose.

Mind should be focussed on the abdominal region. In final position the weight transfer is through toes, knees, chest, hands and chin (eight points). This position in Hindi is named as 'ASHTANGA NAMASKARA.'

Position 7:

To change position from position-6, lower the buttocks and hips on to the floor deeply inhaling while raising the torso and arching the back, straighten the elbows, arch the back and push the chest forward, to imitate the cobra (a deadly Indian snake variety) head pose.

Bend the head back and direct the gaze upward so that the eyes focus on the focal point. The thighs and hips shall remain on the floor and the arms shall keep on providing support to the trunk.

Arms shall remain slightly bent. Only if your spine is very flexible and after attaining mastery over all positions, do try to straighten up arms. Keep mind focussed on providing relief and relaxation to the spine. This position of imitating cobra is known as 'BHUJANGASANA.'

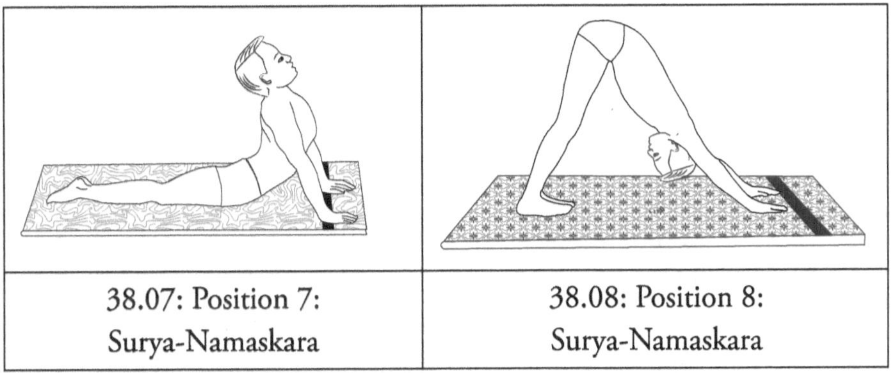

38.07: Position 7: Surya-Namaskara	38.08: Position 8: Surya-Namaskara

Position 8:

The final position in this is a repetition of final position in position-5. From position-7, you need to smoothly transit your posture to position-5. From 'BHUJANGASANA' transfer yourself to 'PARVATASANA.'

The hands and feet do not move, they shall remain as they were, in position-7. Exhale deeply, raise the buttocks and lower the heels to the floor. Keep mind focussed on relaxing the hips or on the throat region. This position as you already know is 'PARVATASANA.'

Position 9:

This stage is also the same as position-4. Inhale while assuming the pose. Keep the palms flat on the floor. Bend the left leg and bring the left foot forward between the hands. At the same time, lower the right knee so that it touches the floor, and push the pelvis forward.

Tilt the head backwards, arch the back and gaze at the focal point. Keep mind focussed on the stretch from the thighs to the chest or on the focal point of all senses. You are transiting from 'PARVATASANA' to 'ASHWA SANCHALANASANA.'

Position 10:

This position is repetition of position-3 ('PADAHASTASANA'). You need to change the body posture from position-9 to position-3. Exhale while performing the movements. Bring the right foot forward, next to the left foot. Straighten both knees. Bring the forehead as close to the knees as possible without over-straining. Keep mind focussed on the pelvic region.

Position 11:

The final position in this, is the same as position-2 ('HASTA UTTHANASANA'). Inhale while straightening the body. Keep the mind focussed on the abdominal stretch and lungs expansions. Raise the torso and stretch the arms above the head. Keep arms separated, shoulder width apart. Bend the head, arms and upper torso backwards.

Position 12:

This is the final position of the first half-cycle of 'Surya-Namaskara' and is the same as Position number 1. Exhale while transiting from Position-11. Bring the palms together in front of the chest and fold hands in 'Namaskar Mudra.' Focus mind on the heart region, the epicentre of all emotions. Meditate for a few seconds.

Position 13 to 24:

The above twelve positions of 'Surya-Namaskara' are to be practised twice to complete one full round of Asana. Positions 1 to 12 constitute the first half of the round.

In the second half the positions are repeated with some changes. When transferring from position 15 to 16, instead of stretching the right foot backwards, stretch the left foot back. In position 21, the right leg will get bent and right foot brought forward between the hands. This means that you need to repeat positions 1 to 12, primarily involving right leg instead of left leg.

Ending Phase:

After completing each half-round, lower the arms to the side, relax the body, closely observe the breathing pattern. See that breathing returns to normal.

On completion of full rounds of 'Surya-Namaskara' lie down in 'Shavasana' for a few minutes. Allow heartbeat, breathing and respiration to return to normal. Relax all muscles.

Day Thirty-Nine: The Yoga Asana in Standing Postures: Part – II

Learning and Practice for the Day

39.01: The Palm Tree Posture: Tadasana

You are already familiar with this Asana. It is included here again to complete the series of Asana in standing postures in proper chronological order. This is the starting and relaxing posture for all Asanas in this series.

Precautions:

Persons suffering from acute cardiac problems, varicose veins and vertigo should avoid lifting the toes in final posture.

Steps:

<table>
<tr>
<td>

Stand with feet 2 to 6 inches apart. Interlock the fingers, inserting fingers of right hand in the hollows between the fingers of left hand.

Turn the wrists outwards. Inhale deeply, raising the arms up and bringing them in line with shoulders, above your head. Palms remaining interlocked should be facing skywards.

</td>
<td>

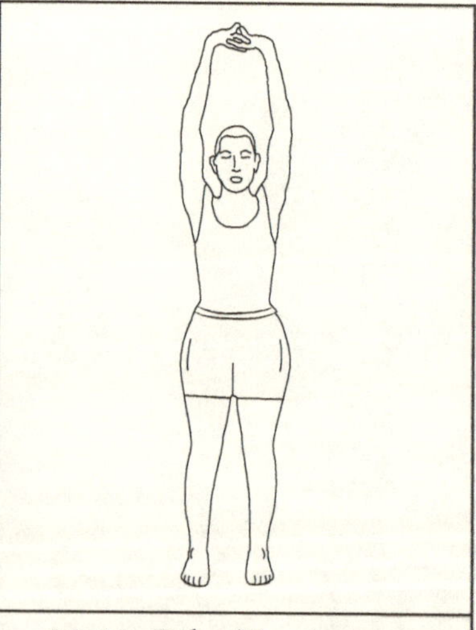

39.01: Palm Tree Posture

</td>
</tr>
</table>

Raise the heels off the floor, maintaining balance and not allowing unnecessary swaying or back and forth movements. Body weight should be uniformly distributed on both feet.

Retain the breath and remain in this posture for ten to fifteen seconds. Exhale normally and bring the arms down. Finally release the interlock of fingers and bring the arms down parallel to the trunk and come back in standing position, i.e., the starting posture. Recollect the correct procedure for relaxing and before proceeding for exercises.

The Hindi word 'Tada' means 'the palm tree' or 'mountain.' This Asana aims to teach one to attain the stability, firmness and deep rootedness of a palm tree/mountain. This is the starting (the base) position for all the standing Asanas.

39.02: The Tree Posture: Vraksha-Asana

Precautions:

The patients suffering from arthritis, vertigo and acute obesity, should not attempt this Asana.

Steps:

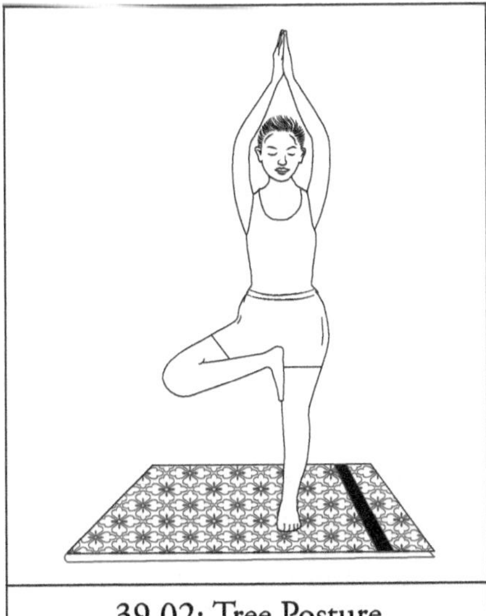

39.02: Tree Posture

Stand with feet 2 to 6 inches apart. Mark a point in the horizon or front wall and focus vision on this point. This is important to ensure maintenance of balance in final posture.

Exhaling deeply, bend the right leg and place the foot on the inside of the left thigh. The heel should be touching or as close as possible to the perineum. Inhaling deeply extend the arms up and join the palms together in 'Namaskar Mudra.'

You are balancing the full body weight on one leg. Body is likely to sway left to right or back and forth. Maintain balance, carefully. Stay in the position for ten to twenty seconds, breathing normally.

Exhale and bring the arms and right foot down. Relax and after five to ten seconds of relaxation repeat the exercise by bending the left leg and maintaining body balance on right leg.

'Vraksha,' the Hindi word means tree. This Asana derives its name from tree as the final position resembles the shape of the tree.

39.03: The Hands to feet posture: PADA-HASTA-ASANA:

The next Asana in this series is 'Hands to feet posture' or 'Pada-Hasta-Asana.' This posture is also referred as 'UTTANA-ASANA.' This is the same as Postion-3 in 'Surya-Namaskara.' You are already familiar with this.

Tip of the Day

Tip: Breath Synchronisation
Breath synchronisation is a very important part of Yoga. It is easy in understanding. But a beginner is likely to face huge issues with this. First issue may be of accurately remembering the correct sequence and second may be of timing the inhalation, exhalation and retention perfectly, to match with the physical part of the exercises. The best way is to initially remember the point, during the physical part of the exercise, where exhalation is prescribed. Cause a forceful exhalation at that point only and allow inhalation and retention to occur naturally. This way, you may with sustained practice, achieve the perfection in synchronisations. This tip is however for beginners only. There is no substitute for a perfectly performed set of physical exercises with breath synchronisation. To understand the difference, you may perform the physical exercise both ways, i.e., with and without synchronisation initially.

39.03: The Half Wheel Posture: ARDHA-CHAKRA-ASANA

Precautions:

In case of vertigo or a tendency to giddiness, avoid this practice. Patients suffering from hypertension should exercise utmost care while bending backwards.

Steps:

Stand with feet together or 2 to 6 inches apart. Provide support to the back, at the waist with all the fingers together pointing either forward or downward.

Drop the head backwards, allowing neck to stretch backwards as far as comfortably possible. Inhaling deeply, bend backwards from the lumbar region. Exhale and relax.

Stay in this posture for ten to thirty seconds, breathing normally. Inhale and slowly come up. Release the tension in neck and bring head in normal position. Release the hand grip and allow hands to hang loosely by the sides of the trunk. Relax.

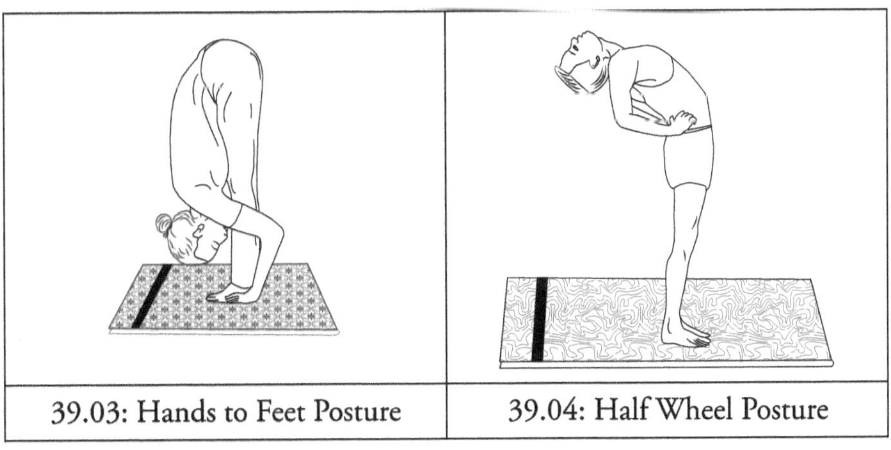

39.03: Hands to Feet Posture	39.04: Half Wheel Posture

39.04: The Triangular Posture: Trikona-Asana

Precautions:

This posture is to be avoided, in case of slipped disc, sciatica and after undergoing abdominal surgery. Do not try to do beyond capacity or overdo the lateral stretch. If it is difficult to touch the feet in final posture, reach up to knees instead.

Steps:

From the starting pose of Tadasana, take feet apart and stand with feet comfortably apart. Slowly raise both the arms sideways till they are horizontal. Slightly twist and bend the torso to allow hands to attain the posture.

Exhaling deeply, slowly bend to the right side and place the right hand just behind the right foot. Grip the leg with hand, if required to maintain balance. The left arm be straight up, in line with the right arm.

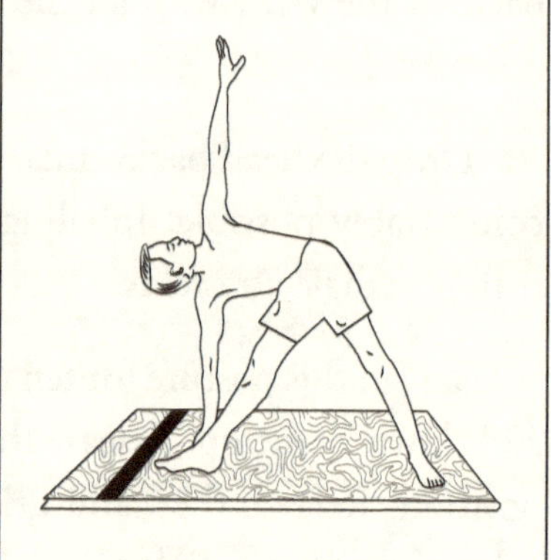

39.05: Triangular Posture

Your body should now resemble a three-armed triangle made by trunk, and the limbs. Try to make a smooth triangle with each arm of triangle in straight lines.

Turn the left palm, held over head, forward. Turn your head upwards and focus eyes and mind at the tip of the left middle finger. Remain in this posture for ten to twenty seconds with normal breathings. Slowly come up inhaling. Rest in Tadasana for a few seconds. Repeat on left side.

'Tri' means 'Three,' 'Kona' means 'Angle,' thus 'Trikona' means 'Triangle.' The Asana derives its name, as the final posture takes the body to a triangular shape.

Chapter–Five

Day Forty: The Yoga Asana in Sitting Postures

Learning and Practice for the Day

Before attempting to learn any asana of this series, you need to refurbish your knowledge of sitting postures particularly Vajrasana (Posture Number S2). Go back to Chapter-One, Day-nine, if required. For Asanas in this series, Sukhasana or Vajrasana is the starting and relaxation posture. You have already learnt a few Asanas of this series. Asana such as Marjari Asana and a few subtle exercises of spinal group were borrowed from this series. We will learn a few more Asanas of this series today.

40.01: Intoxicating Bliss Pose

Steps:

Sit in Vajrasana. Place the palms on top of the heels, such that the fingers are pointing towards each other. If this is found uncomfortable, place the palms just above the heels. Keep the head and spine erect as usual. Close the eyes and relax the whole body. Fix the focus of attention and senses at focal point.

Breathing: be slow and deep. Imagine that the breath is moving in and out of the eyebrow centre. Inhale from the focal point up to the navel region and exhale from the navel region to the focal point. This posture is also called as ANANDA-MADIRASANA.

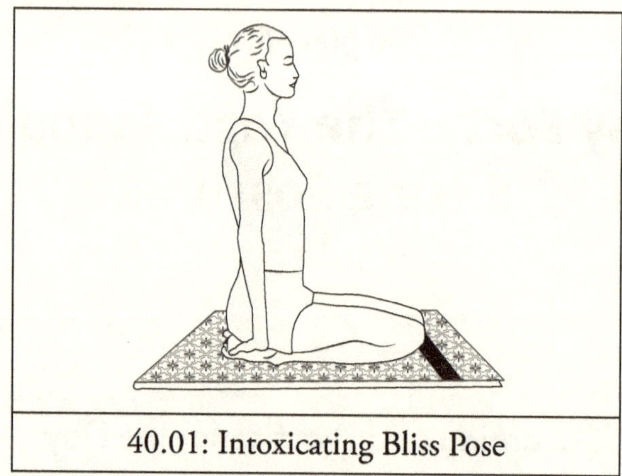

40.01: Intoxicating Bliss Pose

Focus: In the early stages of the practice, physical part of awareness should be on the breathing process. When sufficient relaxation is achieved, awareness may be transferred to the focal point.

Note: The thumbs may press any points on the sole according to specific effects required in the body. For exact details, read some books or seek the advice of someone with knowledge of acupressure, acupuncture or reflexology. Ananda-madirasana may also be performed as an alternative to classical meditation postures.

40.02: Manduk-Asana

Steps:

Sit comfortably in the posture of Vajrasana. Place your right palm over the stomach, fingers remaining below the navel area closely joined. Now place your left palm also above the right palm, thumbs and fingers closely joined together.

Now exhale out completely and shift the upper body in front directions. Legs shall remain joined as they were in Vajrasana. Try to touch the ground with the tip of your nose. Hold the posture for as long as you can comfortably hold it, retaining the breath.

Return to Vajrasana while inhaling forcefully. Relax in Vajrasana.

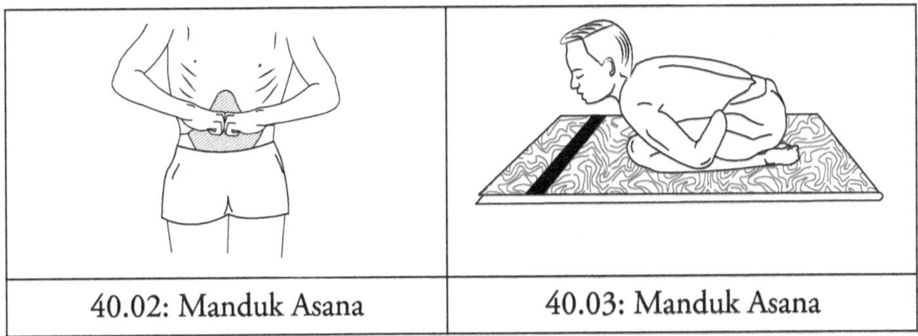

| 40.02: Manduk Asana | 40.03: Manduk Asana |

Variations:

First: Instead of palm, form a close fist, keeping the thumb inside the clenched fist and place both clenched fists close to each other below the navel region. Perform Mandukasana.

Second: Place clenched fist of right hand above navel point covering the point completely and left hand fist above the right hand fist. Perform Mandukasana.

Third: In this version first perform Mandukasana, keeping hands in any one of the positions as above, gain the posture as depicted in 40.02. The nose should be as close to the ground as feasible. Hold the posture, in retention phase of breath, for as long as it is comfortable. When it is no longer comfortable to retain the breath, marginally and very slightly release the tightness of posture. Consciously cause one more attempt at exhalation and final desperate attempt to allow tip of nose to touch the ground. Release the posture as soon as feasible. Relax.

This Asana is beneficial in diabetes and abdominal disorders. For diabetes, keep fist above navel before diaphragm and in case of gastric, constipation etc., keep fist around both sides of navel.

40.03: The Firm/Auspicious Posture: Bhadhra-Asana

This posture is suitable for long comfortable sitting, as for Meditation and Pranayama. 'Bhadhra' means firm or auspicious.

Precautions:

This practice is to be avoided in case of severe arthritis and sciatica.

Steps:

Sit comfortably, keeping spine straight, head high and legs stretched out straight in front. Keep legs comfortably apart. Keep the hands beside the hips, fingers pointed forwards. Arms shall remain slightly bent at elbows, so that the palms may comfortably rest on the ground. Breathe normally. This posture is called 'DANDA-ASANA.'

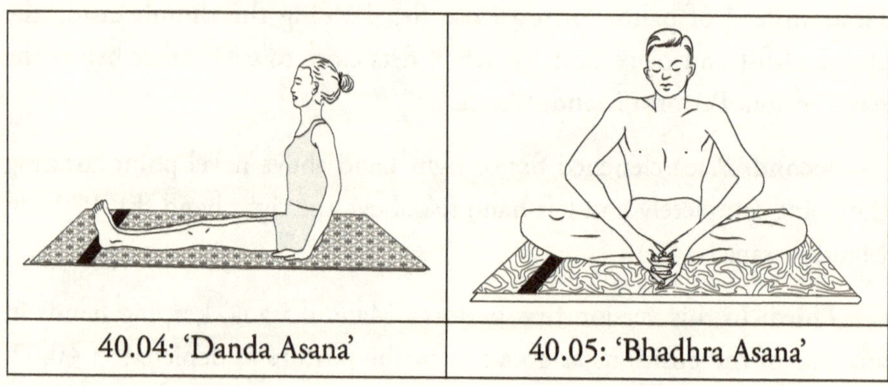

| 40.04: 'Danda Asana' | 40.05: 'Bhadhra Asana' |

Now put the sole of your feet together, toes pointed outwards. Exhale and clasp your hands together on your toes. Pull the heels as close as possible up to the perineum region. Try to touch the floor, with thighs.

The skins of heels and toes should exert massaging/caressing pressure on each other. If your thighs are not touching or are not close to the floor, place a soft cushion underneath the knees for support. This is the final posture of 'BHADHRA-ASANA.' Stay in this posture for some time.

40.04: The Half Camel Posture: Ardha Ustra-Asana

Precautions:

This asana is to be avoided in cases of hernia, abdominal injuries, arthritis, vertigo and pregnancy.

Steps:

Sit in the comfortable base position or Sukhasana. From relaxation posture attain the posture as in 'DANDA-ASANA.' (Legs joined, hands placed beside the hips).

Fold your legs and sit on your heels. Keep the thighs close and big toes touching. Place the hands on the knees. The spine and head should be straight. This, as you know, is 'Vajrasana.' Relax in this posture for a few moments.

Inhaling deeply and smoothly transferring upper body weight upwards, stand on your knees. Place the hands on the waist with fingers pointing downwards. Keep elbows and shoulders parallel.

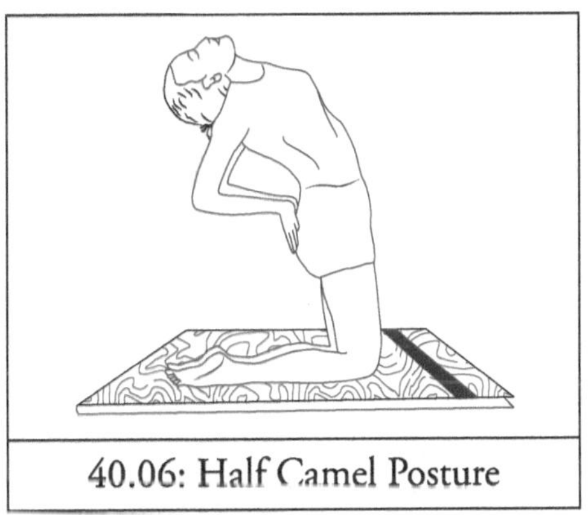

40.06: Half Camel Posture

Now bend the head back and stretch the neck muscles. Inhale and bend the trunk backwards as much as comfortably possible. Exhale and relax! Try and keep the thighs perpendicular to the ground. Remain in this posture for ten to thirty seconds with normal breathing. Inhaling deeply return to Vajrasana. Sit and relax in Vajrasana till breathing is normal.

This Asana derives its name from the hump of the camel. The position of your body in final version of this Asana resembles the hump of a camel. Here only first stage (half) of the Asana has been described. Another 'Asana' similar in nature to this is 'Ustrasana.' 'Ustra' means the barber's knife. If you can reach the heels, you can place your hands on them and bend backwards. This is the final position of 'Ustrasana.'

40.05: The Hare Posture: Sasanka Asana

Precautions:

Not to be practised in case of acute backache. Patients with osteoarthritis of the knees should exercise with proper caution. Such patients may also avoid sitting in Vajrasana.

Steps:

Attain the Vajrasana posture. Sit and relax in Vajrasana. Spread both the knees wide apart, keep both the big toes touching. Keep the palms between the knees.

Exhale and slowly stretch them full length. Bend forward and place the chin on the ground. Keep the arms parallel. Look in front and maintain the posture. 'Sasanka' means hare.

The shape of your body in the final position resembles the shape of a hare. Inhale slowly, release the posture and come up. Exhale and come back to Vajrasana. Stretch your legs back to relaxation asana.

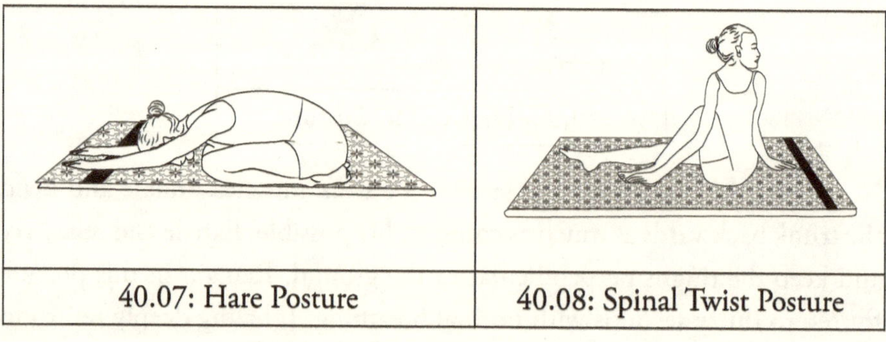

40.07: Hare Posture	40.08: Spinal Twist Posture

40.06: The Spinal Twist Posture: Vakra-Asana

Precautions:

The practise of this Asana is to be avoided in case of severe back pain, vertebral and disc disorders, after abdominal surgery and during menstruations.

Steps:

Attain the posture as in 'Dandasana.' Changing posture from 'Dandasana,' bend the right leg and place the right foot beside the left knee.

Relaxing, twist the upper body, the torso to the right. Now bring the left arm around the right knee and clasp the right big toe or place the palm beside right foot.

Take the right arm back and keep the palm on the ground with the back straight. Remain in this posture for ten to thirty seconds with normal breathing and relax. Take out your hands with exhalation and relax. After a few seconds of relaxation repeat the same exercise on the other side.

Day Forty-One: The Yoga Asana in Lying down Posture

Learning and Practice for the Day

41.01: The Cobra Posture: Bhujanga Asana

Precautions:

Those suffering from hernia or ulcers should not practise this posture. Persons having undergone any abdominal surgical procedure during the last three to four months should not attempt this Asana.

Steps:

Lie down on your stomach as in Makrasana (Prone posture). Rest and relax! Ensure that your weight is uniformly transferring to the ground. Maintain about one foot gap between the legs and feet.

Now to start this Asana, join your legs, stretch your arms, and lift your head slightly up. Fold the right arm and place the right palm beneath the forehead, palm facing downward. Now place left palm over the right palm, left palm also facing downwards, fingers of both palms pointed in directions opposite to each other.

The left palm should completely cover and embrace the right palm. You have thus created a cushion for your forehead to rest on. The weight of your head should be uniformly and smoothly transferring to left palm, from left palm to right palm and from right palm to ground. Rest in this posture for a few seconds.

Stage-1: Retaining the palm-formation as before and after deep inhalation, lift your head, then chin, then neck and thereafter the upper body up to navel, smoothly up, taking head as high as convenient. Raise your head and upper torso just like the cobra (a lethal variety of snakes in India) raises its head. Hands should remain firmly placed, joined as in starting position. Arms shall be raised for supporting the weight of upper body and providing balance. Retain the posture. Breathe normally. Now exhale, come back and place your forehead on the jointed palm formations as before. This was the first stage of easy version called 'Saral Bhujangasana.'

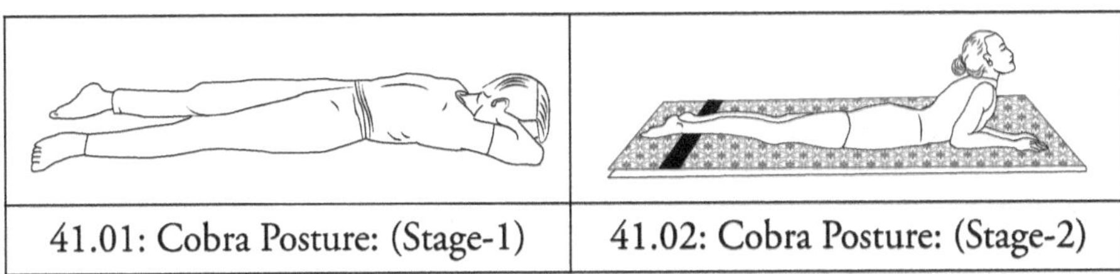

| 41.01: Cobra Posture: (Stage-1) | 41.02: Cobra Posture: (Stage-2) |

Stage-2: Now release the palm formations, place the forehead touching the ground, and place your hands just beside the body, keeping palms facing downwards, and elbows on the ground. Observe and mentally remember the points and positions of your elbows at this juncture. Now inhaling, lift the chin, neck, chest and upper torso up to navel region as in Stage-1. Keep hands firmly on ground, both arms uniformly supporting the upper body weight. Retain the posture. Breathe normally. Now exhale, come back and place your forehead on the ground as before. This was the second stage of easy version called 'Saral Bhujangasana.'

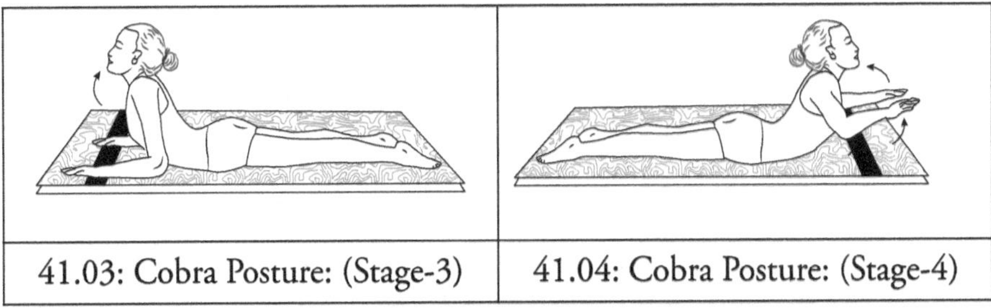

| 41.03: Cobra Posture: (Stage-3) | 41.04: Cobra Posture: (Stage-4) |

Stage-3: Now keep your palms beside the chest, where your elbows were in Stage-2 and raise the elbows. Inhale deeply, lift the chin and chest up to navel region as in Stage – 1 and Stage – 2. Try to straighten your arms at elbows. Arms must uniformly support the upper body's weight. Try and keep the legs firm so that no load or strain is felt on the lumbar spine. This is the first stage of the real 'BHUJANGA ASANA.'

Stage-4: In this stage along with the upper body up to navel region, the hands, initially placed as in Stage-3 shall also be lifted along with the upper body. The weight of the upper body shall transfer through the stomach near the navel region remaining in touch with the ground. This is the second stage of the real 'BHUJANGA ASANA.'

41.02: Shalabh Asana

Precautions:

Cardiac patients and persons with heart related complications should not perform this Asana. In case of severe or mild back pains, perform each step very slowly, carefully and preferably under supervision. Those suffering from high blood pressure, peptic ulcers and hernia should also not attempt this posture.

Note: This Asana is recommended to be performed in sequential manner, immediately after performing Bhujangasana.

Steps:

Lie down flat on your belly (stomach) in Makarasana (Prone Posture). Ensure that body weight is uniformly transferring to floor through as many pressure points as feasible. Place the chin on the floor in resting position. Keep both hands beside the body, palms facing upwards.

Stage-1: Inhale deeply and raise left leg off the floor as much as you can comfortably raise it. Keep the legs straight, stretched and toes pointed, without bending the knees. Extend the arms and legs well to ease the lifting of the body up, off the floor. You may use your palm to support the raised leg. Hold the posture for ten to twenty seconds breathing normally. Exhale and bring the leg slowly down towards the floor. Rest for a few seconds till breathing become normal!

Stage-2: Repeat the same step with the right leg. Rest for a few seconds till breathing becomes normal.

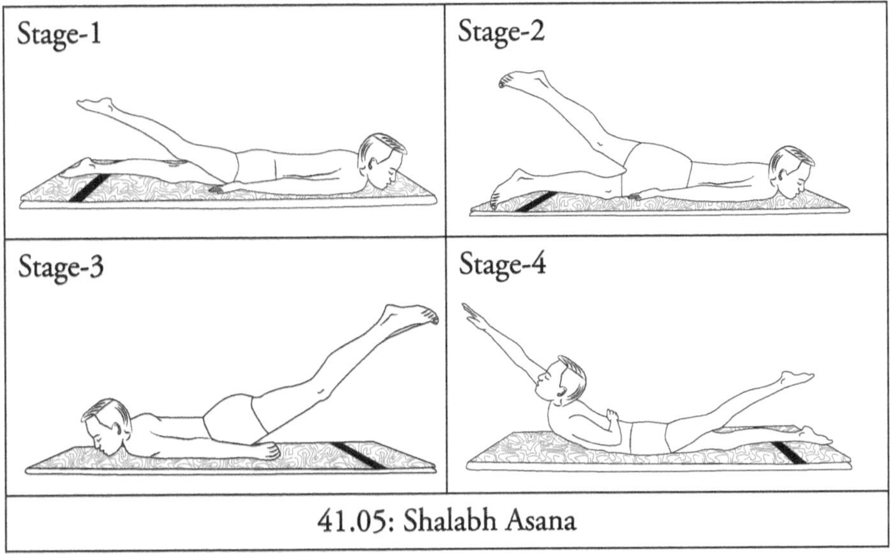

41.05: Shalabh Asana

Stage-3: Repeat the same step raising both legs together. Legs should be as close to each other as feasible.

Stage-4: Some more variations include placing the right hand on the back and lifting the left hand and right leg together. Similarly placing left hand on hips, lift right hand and left leg together. And finally pacing both hands interlocked on hips, lift both legs and head upwards.

Note: To improve the posture, pull the knee caps consciously up and squeeze the buttocks.

Tip of the Day

Tip: Pointed Toes
The importance of pointed toes has already been adequately explained. You need to further understand that in some of the exercises, particularly those involving legs and spinal systems you are pushing, pulling, stretching or rotating the entire muscles and nervous system. It is therefore important that this set of muscles/nerves are firmly held in position at end points. By pointing your toes, you are doing exactly that.
To implement the concept initially in your routine practices is as difficult as it is simple in understanding. To gradually build up the habit of pointing toes, initially make it a habit to check after performing a set of exercises requiring pointed toes, if you have performed it with pointed toes or not. If result of this check is 'negative' or 'don't remember,' repeat the exercise, by consciously and deliberately keeping toes pointed, eyes open and focussed on toes.
In case of difficulty in pointing toes, slightly bend and allow the finger next to the big toes to be placed over the nails in the big toe. This way toe will perforce pull the finger up and remain in pointed state.

41.03: The Bridge Posture: Setu-Bandh-Asana

Precautions:

Not to be performed by persons suffering from ulcers and hernia. Women should not practise this Asana in advanced stage of pregnancy.

Steps:

Lie down in Shavasana. Please note that the head will remain in contact with the floor in the final position of this practice. The posture in the final position is difficult to hold. If required, you may support your body at the waist level with your hands.

Bend both the legs at the knees and bring the heels near the buttocks. Try to touch the heel with hips. While holding both the ankles firmly, keep the knees and feet in one straight line. Inhale deeply and slowly raise your buttocks and trunk up as much as you can. You are required to imitate the formation of a bridge, with your feet and head acting as abutments.

Remain in this position for ten to thirty seconds, breathing normally. Exhale and slowly return to the base position, the 'Shavasana.' Rest and relax in this posture till breathing becomes normal. Do take proper care not to cause any abrupt drop of your back. It may injure the spine. 'Setu,' a Hindi word means 'Bridge.' 'Bandh' is 'to tie' or 'to construct.' 'Setu-Bandh' therefore means 'to erect a bridge.'

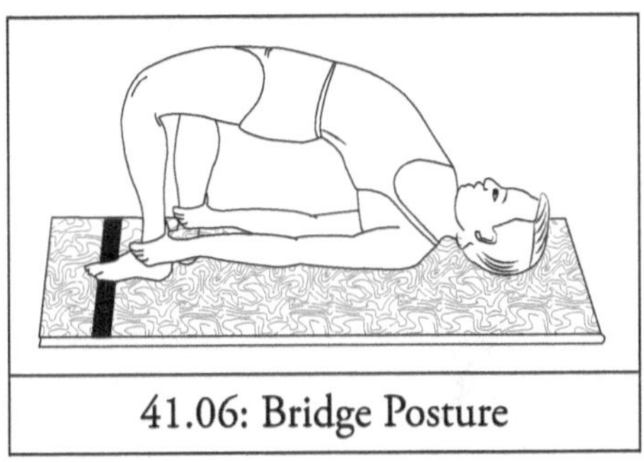

41.06: Bridge Posture

41.04: Markata Asana-Ii

This Asana is the last phase of Sleeping Abdominal Stretch Pose (Chapter-Four, Day-Thirty-three Exercise Number 33.04). This may be performed in conjunction with the referred subtle exercises. It is included separately in this Chapter due to enhanced difficulty level.

Steps:

Lie down in 'Shavasana.' Spread both the arms outwards, keeping palms facing upwards and arms at right angle to the body. Maintain about one foot gap between the legs.

Now lift the left leg, and making a smooth circular movement bring this to the right side as close to the right palm as feasible. Try to touch the right palm with left toe. Simultaneously, move the head to the right side.

If it is difficult to reach the palm of opposite hand with leg, initially allow leg to reach as close to palm in other direction, lift the hand, catch hold of the big toe and pull the leg as down as possible.

Focus and feel the stretch in right hip junction. The muscles and nerves are getting stretched. Keep on holding the breath. Retain the posture till such time as you are comfortable. Slowly bring the right leg back to the original position and head in the central position, face up.

Now repeat the same exercise with right leg, bringing it to left side trying to touch the right palm. Head will go in opposite, i.e., in right direction.

This is one round. You may repeat three to five rounds as per your capacity. Rest and relax in Shavasana.

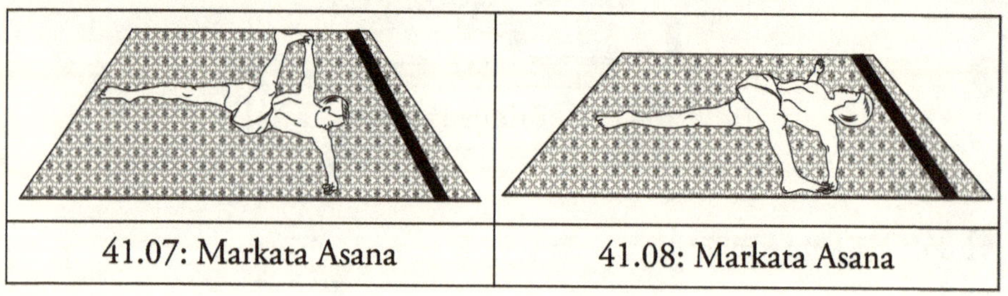

| 41.07: Markata Asana | 41.08: Markata Asana |

Day Forty-Two: Ending Your Daily Yoga Session

Learning and Practice for the Day

Before ending your forty-five + minutes of Yogic routine, the last but one Asana should be as under:-

42.01: Yogic Mantra Recitation Posture

Precautions:

Not to be performed by persons with serious back conditions, back pain, or suffering from any spine/nerve related diseases. This asana is recommended to be performed after completing your daily routine of exercises, as last Asana, before proceeding for final relaxation phase (i.e., Sampoorna Shavasana).

Steps:

Lie down in the starting posture of Shavasana (Supine Posture-Base position) palms down. Keep the eyes closed throughout. Breathe in deeply. Hold the breath and then raise both the legs, taking support of arms, if required. Try to bring legs as upwards as possible, making a 90-degree angle with the ground.

Now raise both hands also upwards. Hands should also make 90-degrees angle with the ground. Both hands and legs shall remain parallel to each other. Hold the posture and recite loudly some mantra.

You may recite 'Gayatari Mantra' or some other mantras of your choice. If you are not comfortable with mantra recitation, count loudly retaining the posture! Retain the posture for as long as you can comfortably retain it.

If it is difficult to keep legs raised upwards, provide support to legs with hands. Count to 120 mentally (or for longer, if possible). Focus of concentration should be at navel point. You may experience some unusual vibrations around the bellybutton. Breathing normally but synchronised with mantra recitation or counting, breathe out and return to the supine position. First bring legs down and thereafter the hands. Be careful not to injure the back of the head, legs and hands while returning to the floor. No abrupt fall, please. Relax the whole body.

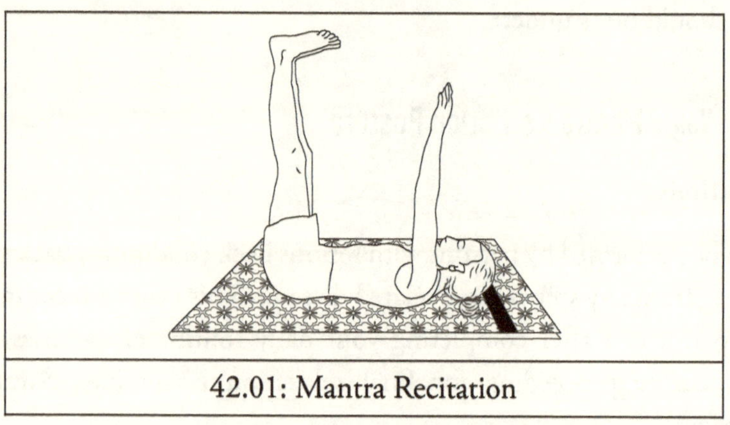

42.01: Mantra Recitation

Relax in Sampoorna Shavasana (the relaxation to be performed after ending the daily routine) after this exercise.

Ending:

Kindly recollect and recall, that I have asked you to look at everything in Yoga from the prism of building up a story, with build-up, climax and ending phases. You have already reached the climax, attained the zenith and climbed Mount Everest with all minor exercises and complex Asanas.

It is now time to come down to mother earth, time to bring your body back to normal state, to shift your focus to routine grinds, tasks, targets and deadlines for the day. And it is time to enjoy the fruits of the sweat and the efforts. You must do this also properly. After completing the last Asana, posture, or routine, you must perform 'Sampoorna Shavasana' (The complete relaxation exercise). Here is how:

42.02: Sampoorna Shava Asana (The Complete Relaxation Exercise)

During your Yoga session, you were asked to attain a perfect posture. You were also asked to stretch or compress some organs. You also rotated some body parts. Though you were asked to take short breaks and relax, that relaxation was primarily to prepare you for the next set of rotations, stretching, compressions and postures. In all these processes, you are likely to build up some tensions, compressions, rotational stresses and strains.

All these residual stresses, strains, tensions and compressions now need to be released and relieved. You also need to allow smooth dissipation of static electrical and excess thermal energies. It is easy; rest in a good relaxation posture, like Shavasana for some time, bring the body to the peace of a corpse and these stresses and strains should disappear. The process gets expedited, if energies of mind and senses are also harnessed in relaxing the body.

But you were also asked to focus your mind and all your senses on some points, some activities. Your senses and mind also experienced the same kinds of stresses and strains. They are not ready for a new task. They also require release, relief and rest. Now, that is difficult.

Allow some freedom and the mind and senses will again start wandering. So! How to relax everything together? The answer lies in Sampoorna Shavasana. To enable your senses and your mind to return to the normal state, the base position, they need to be actively involved in the relaxation, such that they aid and abet the relaxation of body and in turn get themselves relaxed. Sounds complex and difficult. It indeed is difficult, but very, very important.

No matter, how hard I try, I really cannot explain it in narrative form. So, what I request you is to create an audio recording of the following narrations on your Smartphone or any other audio recording device. Play this recording, while lying in Shavasana. Imagine that your 'adopted Guru' is giving you the instructions. Follow the instructions blindly, honestly, diligently and carefully.

If you have any doubts on the efficacy and effectiveness of Sampoorna Shavasana vis-à-vis Shavasana, conduct a simple experiment. After conducting an intense forty-five+ minutes of Yogic exercises, just perform Shavasana for five to ten minutes for two to three days. Repeat the same for two to three days with performing Sampoorna Shavasana in the end. See the difference.

You are likely to feel tiredness or may be mild pains in some limbs in the first instance. So! Take my advice seriously. Do end your session properly with complete set of Sampoorna Shavasana. Here goes the narration that you need to record and play, while lying in Shavasana.

"Now, we are going to perform a very important Asana. The Sampoorna Shavasana. Listen to my instructions carefully, listen to each and every word very carefully and follow my instructions honestly. Surrender yourself to me. Relax! Relax! And Relax! Relax your body! Relax your mind! Relax your heart! Relax your soul! Relax! Relax! And Relax!

Lie down comfortably on your back. Allow the weight of your body to be uniformly transferring to ground. Let there be no undue pressure point in smooth weight transfer to ground. Tilt your head slightly to the right. Keep your hands about one foot away from your body. Keep Left hand on left side and right hand on right side. Hands should be loose, palms facing upwards, fingers loosely resting. Palms should be half open and half closed.

Let there be about one foot distance between your legs. Allow legs to relax. Leave them free to relax. Leave them loose. Release the pointed toes. Relax the toes. Let there be no stretching in any of the body parts.

Place your tongue behind the lower jaw line pressing the roots of teeth line and gums supporting teeth. Breathe through the mouth normally! Use the air passage above tongue for breathing. Breathe normally through mouth. Allow your nostrils to relax. Relax! Relax and Relax! Leave all parts of the body loose. Leave the complete body loose! Enjoy the peace of a corpse. Let there be some smile on your face. Enjoy! Enjoy! And Enjoy! Relax! Relax! And Relax!

Now I instruct you to keenly observe all the organs and parts of your body, one by one, as per my instructions. Talk to the organs and ask them to relax, to loosen up and to enjoy. We will traverse the body, covering all parts, one by one, from top to bottom, from head to toes and then from down to up. Focus your mind on the focal point of your senses. As soon as I pronounce the name of the organ, take your mind to that organ, shift focus on that organ, talk to the organ, loosen it up, and relax it!

First, we will travel inwards, through inside the body. Follow me carefully. Follow my instructions honestly. Shift focus to the organ, talk to the organ, relax it, and loosen it up. Imagine that a miniature version of you has entered inside your body and is able to clearly see, feel and converse with your internal organs. We are travelling inside your body from head to toe.

Left brain! Relax! Creative brain, Relax! Relax! And Relax! Loosen up! Loosen up! Loosen up!

Right brain! Relax! The Logical, Mathematical brain, Relax! Relax! And Relax! Loosen up! Loosen up! Loosen up! Right brain, please ask all body parts to relax!

Complete brain! Head and Skull! Relax! Relax! Relax! And Relax! Loosen up! Loosen up! Loosen up! Slacken up! Slacken up!

Slacken up! Let there be no thoughts and no clutter in your mind. Relax your mind! Relax!

Now come to the eyes! Look at the optic nerve, the retina, the lenses, the pupils, the eyelids! Look how beautiful they are! Leave your eyes loose; leave the retina, the pupils, and the eyelids loose. Loosen up your eyes! Relax! Relax! And Relax!

Now shift the focus of your attention to your ears! Look at the auditory nerve, the stirrups, the eardrums, the ear canal, and the flaps! How obedient, how subservient they are! Leave your ears loose! Loosen up your ears! Relax! Relax! And Relax!

Now relax your tongue, your teeth, your gums and your jaws! Relax! Relax! And Relax!

Now keenly observe your heart! Look how smoothly, how beautifully it is working! Look at the rhythm! Look, all pumps, all valves and all veins are so neat and so clean. They are working beautifully. Relax! Relax! And Relax! Relax your Heart! Loosen up your Heart! Slacken up your Heart! Cool down your heart! Calm down! Relax! All is well! All is well! All is well! So, Relax!

Look at your kidneys, look at your lungs. Look at the liver. Look how good they are looking! How good they are feeling! Enjoying! Relax! Relax! And Relax! Relax Your Lungs! Relax Your Kidneys! Relax your liver! Relax! Relax! And Relax!

Look at the Gallbladder, the Pancreas, the small intestines, and the large intestines! Look how fresh, happy and healthy they are looking. Having soaked so much of oxygen, they are all rejoicing. Relax them up. Loosen all parts of the lower body! Loosen your stomach! Slacken your belly. Relax! Let all body parts be at rest, loose, with no tension and no stress. Relax!

Relax your hip junctions! Relax your leg junctions! Relax your hips! Relax! Relax! And Relax! Relax your thighs! Relax your knees!

Relax your ankles! Relax your feet! Relax your toes! Relax! Relax! And Relax! Loosen up all joints, and all junctions! Relax your legs! Relax! Relax! And Relax! Relax your legs! Relax the complete lower body. Relax! Relax! And Relax!

Now we will similarly travel inwardly from toe to head. Look at your toes, Relax. Look at the ankle joint. Loosen up! Relax! Look at the knee joints! Loosen up! Relax! We are travelling inwards inside your body. Look at each organ carefully. See there is no stretching, no compressions left. Release all tensions, all compressions. Relax! Relax! And Relax!

Now you will traverse your body outwardly from down to up, from toe to head. Do as I say, sincerely and with complete focus of mind.

Relax your toes! Relax your feet! Relax the ankles! Loosen down everything! Slacken every organ! Relax your knees! Relax your legs! Relax your thighs! Relax the hip junctions! Relax the leg junctions! Relax all joints! Relax the lower body. Check that there is no tension! No stress! No pain! Relax everything!

Relax your back and stomach together. Keenly observe the navel area. Focus your mind, all your senses and all your awareness on the navel region. Relax! Loosen down your body. Check that the body weight is uniformly spread and is uniformly transferring to the ground.

Buddham Sharnam Gacchami!

Anandam Sharnam Gacchami!

Guruwar Sharnam Gacchami!

Relax! Relax! And Relax! Relax your chest! Relax your neck! Relax your chin! Relax your face! Relax your cheeks! Relax your eyes! Relax your forehead! Relax! Relax! And Relax!

Relax your forehead! Relax your Head! Have one closer look at your body! Loosen every organ! Slacken everything! If you are not able to feel comfort placing your neck and head on right side, you may shift it on left side, if that is more comfortable. You must sincerely involve your mind and heart into this relaxation. If any residual stretch or stress is left, in any organ, that organ may cause pain. It may give you lots of discomfort throughout the day. So please do this seriously.

Now I am bringing a magical sieve! Believe my words. I am having a sieve that will filter all the stresses, all impurities, all diseases and all disorders from your body! I will guide you, hold the long handle and pass your body through this sieve!

By the blessings of the creator and the magical powers of Guru, all ills, all stress, all impurities, all diseases and all disorders will get filtered. They will remain on one side of the sieve. And your pure, disease-free and stress-free body will lie here.

Do as I say. Look I am bringing the sieve! Lift your head slightly and allow the sieve to pass through, now lift your neck, lift your shoulders, and allow the sieve to pass through, lift the upper body, lift your legs, and lift your feet. Okay I have filtered your body through this sieve.

Look, there is this blackish substance in this sieve. Now I am going to throw all this muck away. I will clean the sieve. I will now pass your body again through this sieve from toes to head! Lift your body slightly up and allow the sieve to pass through! Look, here I am going upwards taking the sieve. Lift your body slightly upwards from leg to head to allow the sieve to pass through. There are again some very little black substances, in this sieve, I am throwing it away. Now rest assured, be certain, that your body is now clean, pure and free from all disorders.

Your body has now become very light in weight, as all impurities have been filtered out. All dust and dirt have been removed. Look, it is very light now! It has become so light that your body weight has disappeared.

You are as light as the shredded cotton! You are as light as feathers! You are like feathers! You have now got wings and feathers, like birds.

You are floating in the air. You are flying like birds in the sky. You are floating like drones in the sky.

Look at the stars in the sky. It is early morning, there are still a few stars in the sky. Look how brightly they are shining. Look at the mighty mountains, the oceans, the lakes, and the beautiful waterfalls below. Look at the flowers. How beautiful and how fragrant they are!

Look how lucky you are, you are seeing this wonderful scene from up here in the sky. Marvel at the beauty of the nature. Soak in the beauty of nature. Honestly imagine that you are floating in the air, you are flying. Enjoy the moments! Enjoy the bliss! Feel the vibes!

Now imagine that you are slowly coming down, still floating in the air, enjoying a beautiful natural lakeside sight below you, with mountains in the backgrounds and a valley full of flowers of all kinds, all colours on one side, a waterfall complementing and adding to the grandeur and the scenic beauty of the ground waiting for your arrival.

You are now lying amidst this beautiful landscape. The love of your life, the man/woman you will die for, is lying beside you. Feel the love. Feel the romance. Calm your body! Relax! Relax! And Relax!

Buddham Sharnam Gacchami!

Anandam Sharnam Gacchami!

Guruwar Sharnam Gacchami!

Relax! Relax! And Relax!

Relax your body!

Relax your mind!

Relax your heart!

Relax your soul!

Aum Shanti, Shanti, Shanti.”

While the above soundtrack was playing in the background, you were expected to blindly, diligently, honestly and sincerely follow, as instructed, while keeping your body, heart, mind, soul, senses and all awareness in harmony. If you had followed the instructions, your body should be in a relaxed, refreshed and rejuvenated shape.

Shift your complete body weight smoothly on right or left side. Get up taking support of your hands, if required. Palm your eyes. Massage your face. Now massage gently all parts of the body from head to toes and from toes to head.

Bring a positive thought; something concerning the larger pictures, the nature, the environment, the world peace, eradication of hunger, poverty, war, superstitions, violence from this world, to mind. Keep and retain this thought, throughout the day.

It is better if this thought is in the form of some mantra, song, poetry or similar form. You may recite or sing it loudly. Even during the day, if you feel stress, depression, distractions, feel anger, anxiety, fear, or notice aimless wandering of the mind/thoughts, bring your mind to this thought. Better still, sing it loud and clear, enjoying it.

Come on Man! You are now ready to conquer the world!

Day Forty-Three: Create Your Own Package for Daily Practice

Learning for the Day

Now, that you have already created your own package of the Mediation-Pranayama Exercises (your own stress buster), you have already decided the package of Minor Exercises (Sukshma-Vyayama) to be practised daily (with some variations for added variety) on working days in a week and on weekend days and holidays. All that is left is to sprinkle some more Asanas from this Chapter to two of your existing packages, like salt and pepper on your dish, and your complete package is ready.

I hardly have anything more to add to this wisdom, except to make some suggestions to facilitate the process. My suggestions are:

Try to squeeze in and devote as much time as you can spare, early in the morning. Ideally your complete daily Yoga session should initially be for about ninety minutes. This must include fifteen minutes of final relaxation and cooling down phase (ending the session with Sampoorna Shavasana) (refer Chapter-Five), fifteen minutes of Meditation-Pranayama in the beginning of the session and four to five minutes of Pranayama ('Kapala-Bhati,' two to three minutes of slow, soundless breathing outs, and slow 'Anuloma-Viloma' Pranayama for two to three minutes), (refer – Chapter-One to Three), twenty-five to thirty-five minutes of Sukshama-Vyayama (Pawanmukta Series of Asanas, covering all organs from toe to head) (refer Chapter – Four) and fifteen to twenty minutes of Asanas (refer Chapter-Five).

Once you attain reasonable proficiency, start achieving posture quickly and do not require long breaks for relaxations in between two practices/ routines, you may reduce the time to sixty minutes, proportionately reducing time of all sub-sections. Do not neglect the ending section. Ensure to achieve complete relaxed state before leaving your Yoga mat.

You need to access your needs, aims and objectives properly and accurately and fine-tune the timings of sub-sections accordingly. If emotional stresses are of most concern, devote more time to Meditation-Pranayama sections.

If suffering from some lifestyle related diseases (e.g., High Blood Sugar levels, Blood pressure, back pains, poor eyesight, obesity, etc.), devote more time on Asanas having curative effects on these diseases.

Consult a Yoga Expert or an Ayurvedic Medical practitioner or study a good Yoga book on curative aspects of Yoga to choose the Asanas having profound effects on your disease group. Do not ignore the minor exercises. Your daily routine must include one minor exercise for each organ from toe to head. You may not be able to complete all Exercises/Asanas of a series, given the time constraints. It is okay to skip a few in between.

If the duration of your daily practices is anything more than forty-five minutes, take a weekly rest. It is better to take rest on working days, rather than on holidays. Devote holidays to health and happiness, rather than to laziness. If your session timing is just fifteen minutes of Pranayama-meditation (do not feel offended, if someone calls you lazy!), no weekly rest is required. I know, you will somehow find an excuse for weekly rests. No matter what my advice is.

Bring in day-to-day variations. If you decide on just one set of easy-looking or difficult ones (depending on your aptitude), you are more likely to get bored, repeating the same set every day. So, better make six separate sets. One each for each working day (five), and one for holidays. Variations add spice to life. Cut down on spices in food and add those spices here.

Before leaving your Yoga mat, do not forget to bring, keep and retain a good positive thought in your mind. Also, gently and firmly massage all body parts, i.e., legs, hands, belly, back, chest, neck, face and skull. That brings freshness and rejuvenation to body. Spend two minutes on laughter Yoga. You may also recite a mantra.

Last but not the least! Do not leave your Yoga mat till you are certain, beyond doubt that the complete body is fully relaxed and there is no residual stress, strain, stretch and compression left in any of the body parts. Feel refreshed after the session and not drained out and fatigued.

Day Forty-Four: The Yogic Way of Life

Learning for the Day

I had in earlier parts of this guide, waxed eloquent, to coax and cajole you into adopting 'the Yogic way of life.' But, what is this 'Yogic way of life'? Is it just to practise Yoga, routinely performing meditation, Pranayama, and Asanas? Or is it adopting those eight limbs of 'Ashtanga-Yoga'? Or is it imitating those 'Hath-Yogis,' who stand on one foot or on their head, sometimes for years together?

Frankly speaking, I was greedy so far. I was saving the worst for the last. Worst? Why? I mean, people normally save their best for the last. Why save the worst for the last? Well, this part is certainly the best, but it is best only for you, the reader. If you may adopt, even a fraction of what I am going to preach here, it may completely transform your life.

The problems are for me. Firstly, preaching is a difficult task, much more difficult than teaching. There is no new learning involved in this. You know it already, what I am going to tell you here. You may, in fact, know much more about these issues, than I.

Secondly, one cannot bring in convictions in his preaching, unless he practises what he preaches. Honestly, I am still struggling in adoption of what I intend to preach here. Such are the trappings of one's own emotions, lifestyles, the markets, and the society.

It is difficult to unshackle these and live your life the way you know very well, is the correct way of living. So, you and I are together in this boat. Let us sail together. I will try my level best to row this boat as smoothly as possible. But you should know the weather is rough and your boatman is weak.

The question, 'What is the Yogic way of life?' needs to be answered in two contexts.

First, what has been preached in ancient text books and is the universal and the immortal wisdom.

Second, extrapolating those time-tested, universally-accepted concepts of ideal or good ways of living, into modern times, can we derive some inspirations, some new innovative concepts, and adopt them in our lives, for our betterment? Let us explore both.

The conventional wisdom of Yoga:

The widely acknowledged Yogic practices ('Yoga-sadhanas') are: 'Yama,' 'Niyama,' 'Asana,' 'Pranayama,' 'Pratyahara,' 'Dharana,' 'Dhyana,' 'Samadhi,' 'Bandhas' and 'Mudras,' 'Shatkarmas,' 'Yuktahara,' 'Mantra-japa,' and 'Yukta-karma,' etc.

'Yamas' (restraints) and 'Niyamas' (observances) are prerequisites for further Yogic practices. Non-violence ('Ahimsa'), Truth ('Satya'), Not-stealing ('Asteya'), Self-control and un-selfishness are important sub-sets of 'Yamas.' And cleanliness, contentment, greatness of efforts, self-exploration, and faith are important sub-sets of 'Niyama.'

'Asanas,' capable of bringing about stability of body and mind, involve adopting various psycho-physical body patterns and giving one an ability to maintain a body position (a stable awareness of one's structural existence) for a considerable length of time.

'Pranayama' consists of developing awareness of one's breathing, followed by wilful regulation of respiration as the functional or vital basis of one's existence. It helps in developing awareness of one's mind and helps to establish control over the mind.

In the initial stages, this is done by developing awareness of the 'flow of in-breath and out-breath' through nostrils, mouth and other body openings, its internal and external pathways and destinations. In advanced stages, this phenomenon is modified, through regulated, controlled and monitored inhalation leading to the awareness of the body space getting filled, the space or spaces remaining in a filled state, and getting emptied during regulated, controlled and monitored exhalation.

'Pratyahara' indicates withdrawal of one's consciousness from the sensory organs, which connect with the external objects. 'Dharana' indicates broad based field of attention, inside the body and the mind, which is usually understood as concentration.

'Dhyana' (meditation) is contemplation, i.e., focussed attention inside the body and mind, and 'Samadhi' is integration. 'Bandhas' and 'Mudras' as you know are practices associated with 'Pranayama' and 'Meditation.' They are viewed as the higher Yogic practices that mainly adopt certain physical gestures along with control over respiration. These two together, further facilitate control over mind and pave the way for a higher Yogic attainment. However, practice of 'Dhyana,' which moves one towards self-realisation and leads one to transcendence, is considered the essence of 'Yoga Sadhana.'

'Ṣaṭkarmas' are detoxification procedures that are clinical in nature and help to remove the toxins accumulated in the body. 'Yuktahara' advocates appropriate food and food habits for healthy living.

In 'Mantra-Japa,' 'Japa' is the meditative repetition of a mantra or a divine consciousness. 'Mantra-Japa' produces positive mental tracts, helping us to gradually overcome stress. 'Yukta-karma' advocates right karmas or actions for a healthy living.

Extrapolation of the conventional wisdom of Yoga for modern times:

Here are my two-cents-worth efforts, in attempting to extrapolate the spirit of the ancient Yogic principles into the modern age:

Table of the Day

'Yama'	:	The laws of Nature, Universal/International laws, The United Nation Charters, The Human and Animal rights, Sustainable developments.
'Niyama'	:	The set of ideal/desirable human emotions, conducive for betterment of environment, Nation, Society, family, the fellow human beings and the quest for knowledge.
'Dharna' 'Dhyana' and 'Samadhi'	:	To look beyond oneself at the larger pictures of universal peace, humanity, knowledge, wellbeing, eradication of hunger, poverty, illiteracy, and superstition. To make some contributions towards these issues ignoring the personal interests and selfishness. To uplift oneself beyond the physical, mental and emotional boundaries, to be able to contribute for achievements of larger desirable objectives.
'Ahimsa'	:	Vegetarianism. Animal rights. Treating all form of lives and inhabitants of the planet Earth as equal.
Some more	:	Add 'digital' in all the concepts of space. Add 'social media profiles' in all concepts of 'souls' or horizons of life. First, add 'internet,' 'information technology,' 'smart phones,' 'social media,' 'space travels,' 'satellites' and similar existing advanced technologies, and thereafter extrapolate this set for probable future advancements in technologies and human capabilities to complete the picture.

I really do not know where I am heading? And how to wind this up? This topic is so vast. You may find thick books written by learned, enlightened souls on this subject. These books describe just the philosophy of Yoga and Yogic living, without even mentioning techniques or steps of a single 'Asana' or 'Pranayama.'

So, I am adopting some short-cuts here. I am now handing over the oars, the sculls, the rudder and everything else that is available in this boat, to you. I am leaving you with just a few questions for you to answer, while I sit back, relax and enjoy.

You are continuously taking something from the environment. Let us call this as set 'X.' Air, water, space, shelter and such other things, primarily needed for your survival is set 'X.' Yes, I know these are needed for your survival. I am not accusing you of being greedy or exploitative.

You are also returning something back to the environment. Some of which is desirable, e.g., planting trees, and some of which are undesirable, i.e., your liquid, solid and non-bio-degradable wastes. Let us call these sets 'Y' and 'Z' respectively. Now can you demonstrate some mathematical skills and compare the two sets of 'X + Z' and 'Y.' You know what I mean. So, why elaborate further?

Now, please substitute the word 'environment' sequentially with words, 'Nation,' 'State,' 'Municipality,' 'Society' and 'Family' in the above question and solve it again. Hey, share the answers, if your set 'Y' is larger than set 'X + Z,' else you know what needs to be done.

Coming back to how adoption of Yogic way of life can change your life, ponder over a few more issues. Do you think 'common cold' should really be that 'common'? After all, it is just a minor infection in the nose, sinuses and upper respiratory tracts, caused due to minor increases in temperatures and presence of dust, pollens, bacteria and viruses associated with seasonal variations.

These are normal variations, mostly occurring three to four times in a year. And there is supposed to be something called 'immunity,' in your body. It is supposed to fight these viruses by producing 'mucus.'

But go to any chemist, in any change of season and the major contributor to the buzzing cash box and the bulging bank balance is 'common cold.' Jeanie Lerche Davis in the year 2003, estimated the cost of common cold in terms of cure and loss of productivity, for USA alone, to be 40 Billion dollars. The 'commonality' of 'common cold' is because the 'common people' have 'commonly' killed the 'commonly available' immunity, thus exhibiting most 'un-common sense.'

The lure of cure ensures giving a go-by to the prevention, whereas, just ten to fifteen minutes of everyday 'Pranayama' not only ensures prevention and cure of this common menace, but also develops the body's immunity to fight with the brothers and sisters of this 'common cold.' Now the questions.

Can you really trust the great pharmaceutical industry, which cannot even prevent as common a disease as common cold, with your health and wellbeing? And what about cure? Most over-the-counter (OTC) and prescription drugs, do nothing beyond drying up the mucus in the respiratory tract and leaving it there, dried, leeched and waiting for the next attack of viruses or removal.

Similarly, take constipation, irregular bowel movements and similar routine digestion related disorders. Why should they occur? According to doctors, it is not a medical condition. They will also advise you that the key to good health lies in clearing the bowels every day.

We can avoid many diseases and disorders, if we eat proper and clear proper. They will not hesitate in helping you out with costly medicines, for which your system will soon develop immunity and demand more and costlier medicines. All this just because we are so busy that we can't spare thirty out of 1440 minutes (2%) for ourselves.

After acquisition of diseases only, doctors will invariably educate you that diabetes, blood sugar, back pain, high/low blood pressures, etc. are neither diseases nor disorders.

These are simply manifestations of Newton's third law of nature. These are equal and opposite reactions of your body to your actions, fancily named as 'lifestyle-disorders.' So, take Newton and his laws on your side. Give forty-five minutes of good actions. Leave the rest to Sir Newton and his laws.

Do you really believe that those colognes/fragrances/deodorants/scents/perfumes aggressively sold in the market, will make girls/guys fall prey to your charms?

Do you believe that your skin colour will change to bright, white and glowing, with the use of those fairness beauty creams? And that you need all those shampoos, conditioners, dyes, colours and pigments to make your hair, the most useless and worthless part of your appearance, persona and halo, attractive?

Are you convinced that you need all those soaps, body-lotions, moisturisers, shower-gels, face-wash, face-packs and what-nots, to keep your face and body healthy? Do you acquire your wisdom from advertising and markets?

Believe me; the greatest distortions in your life are caused by these two demons. The bests of brains are working for advertising, marketing, selling, fleecing you of your hard-earned wealth, and in turn, giving you false hopes, unwanted aspirations, envies, jealousies, and above all stresses. If you can conquer the market, and make it your slave, you have won half the battles of life.

And it doesn't require much. Allow your sweat, respiration and natural evaporation once in a day. Perform meditation, Pranayama, palming, face massage, allow your arms to caress your cheeks whenever rotating them, and your face will acquire the most beautiful glow, without any need of those chemical-laced cosmetics.

Use a thin cotton/muslin cloth to gently rub your body, three to four times, while bathing. No soap is needed. Soap-operas will also die with soaps. Accept yourself the way you are. Take pride in being what you are. Associate the greys in your hair with wisdom and experience. And, you will transfer all your stresses to the market selling you all these crutches. Enjoy living naturally, in harmony with nature and not in sync with the market.

Allow me to end this section, by leaving you with a few more bullet-points, so that I can heave a real huge sigh of relief.

❖ Accept yourself the way you are and cut down your dependence on fashion, fabric, textiles and cosmetics industry.

❖ Take adequate care of your body, adopt Yoga or make some other fitness regime, improve your dietary habits, and thus cut down on medicine, healthcare and medical-insurance costs.

❖ Accept the family, society and the Governments, the way they are. If possible, make some contributions to make them better. Do not allow these to pass on any parcel of stress to you. Make your life stress-free.

❖ Grow organically some fractions of your food needs, converting the organic waste into compost and thus reap the benefits of good health and reduced food costs.

❖ Live in harmony, rather than in conflict with Nature. Nature will shower her blessings on you.

❖ Cut down your negative set of emotions of ego, jealousy, over-ambition, etc. Attain peace.

❖ Insulate yourself from the negativities, deliberately served in high dosages, in the formats of tragedies, tear-jerkers, negative news, etc. by the entertainment industry and Media (all press, print, electronic, social included), and thus make your life free from these unwanted pains and stresses.

❖ Deliberately inject some more smiles, some more of laughter into your daily consumptions. Life shall be much more beautiful.

❖ Allow your cravings and the creativity, the creative freedom that they seek.

❖ AND FINALLY, be wise enough to make your own do's and don'ts in life for its betterment, rather than being guided by ignorant fools and idiots, like yours truly.

Day Forty-Five: Concluding Remarks

Okay!

Boys and Girls! Ladies and Gentlemen!

It is now time to end the forty-five days' long journey. It is also time for me to make some honest confessions. I might have bragged, boasted and tried to convince you that I will teach you Yoga.

I also wrote a section 'My Pledge-My Promise' making some tall claims. It was all a big prank, a big joke, a huge April-fool kind of joke. I am a cheat, a crook and a big prankster. I couldn't teach you Yoga. Remember! I told you that there are 84,00,000 Asanas. I haven't properly covered eighty-four of them. I do not even know all of them.

All that I have done and accomplished so far, is to awaken you, the atheists, the rationalists, the logical thinkers, and the ones of scientific temperament, from your deep slumber. I have succeeded in cajoling, prodding and prompting you, and was holding your hand up to the gates of the 'Nursery of Yoga.'

I have also tried my level best to convince you to adopt Yoga in your daily lives. Your time to learn Yoga begins now! Your time to start practising Yoga, your own Yogic routines, begins now! My teaching ends here. Your learning process begins now! The last task left for me is to just make two more requests to you.

Start Learning Yoga!

Yoga consists of a huge body of works, left for us as inheritance by our ancestors. Keeping the basic threads intact, the Gurus, the observers, the experimenters, the scientists, the medical professionals, the Yoga practitioners, the enlightened ones and the marketers, all have made huge contributions, making it a very finely knit huge and beautiful canvas.

It is your time to start making the best use of this canvas. Pick up your brush and start painting. It is a huge ocean. The more you swim, the more you will learn. Learning is a never-ending process. Only corpses need not learn anything more.

Start Practising Yoga!

You should have, by now, created your own package of Asanas/ Exercises for daily practice. Be faithful and loyal to your creation. Practise your routines on daily basis without failures.

Pick up any good book on Yoga or ask any teacher. The writer or the teacher will tell you that you will see results of your toil, your sweat, and your efforts, only after six months of regular practice. Show patience! Be pragmatic! Be generous to yourself! Give yourself some time! You will see some results after 145 days of your sustained practice. And, this is not a prank.

Tip of the Day

Tip: Contingency Plans
No matter howsoever sincere you are, in your determination to adopt Yoga, a few issues that will arise in between you and your routine practising of pre-set Yogic exercises are: 'I am not in good mood today,' 'I will start regular practice from tomorrow,' 'Yesterday was too hectic, can't spend one hour for Yoga today, will think tomorrow,' 'I took so much time today to get a clean belly and bowels, can't do Yoga today, will do it regularly from tomorrow,' etc. etc.

Let me assure you that tomorrow will never come. 'Tomorrow' will be in no way different from 'today.' To reinforce your resolve, you may prepare an alternative contingency plan. This contingency plan may include exercises like 'Pranayama during walking' (Refer Day-Twenty) or 'Subtle exercises in standing postures' (Refer Day Thirty-Five) or one or more of 'Packaged stress busters' (Refer Day Twenty-one and Day Twenty-two). Whenever such or similar issues arise in your mind, tell yourself, "Okay, today I am not doing Yoga, will start routinely doing it from tomorrow, for today let me be content with performing my alternative set."

Trust me, if you persist with this, your body and mind will automatically propel you towards the Yoga mat.

It will be still better, if you may create more than one contingency plan. One for each type of foul mood or type of excuse. Allow your mood and mind to throw as many tantrums to you as they like. Your armour of contingency plans will keep you united with your Yoga. Remember, Yoga is all about unity and affinity. Show as much love, affection and addiction to it, as to your loved ones. You cannot even imagine what all you may receive back from Yoga as dividends, for your love and affection.

Welcome to a Healthy, Happy, Peaceful, Stress-free life!

Welcome to THE Yogic Way of Life!

Post Script

"Hey! What happened to that Resume that Photo-Physio-Psychological-Bio-Data, that Physio-Emotional matrix that you made us create?"

Oh! Yes! Thanks for reminding me.

Here is what you are supposed to do with that:

After 145 days of your honest and sincere efforts at adopting a Yogic way of life, after sustained efforts of routinely performing your own package of daily practices, I request you to compare your present state, i.e., your physical, emotional and psychological profiles with your 190 (145 + 45) days old profile. Compare and look for the following changes:

- Is your face profile, the skin texture, the glow on the face, the skin colour and the halo around you, the same as before? Are there some changes? Are these Positives or Negatives?

- Is your body language, the way of walking, the way of climbing stairs and the way of sitting at your desk, table, work-station, or in that corner-cabin the same as before? Are there some changes? Positives or Negatives?

- Are there some changes in your smiling, laughing, thinking patterns, or creativity – cravings? Are there some changes in your feelings about others, the colleagues, the family members, the boss, the environment, nature, the state, the Government or such other things? Are these changes for the better or for worse?

- Is your emotional state and the Emotional Quotient (EQ) the same as before? Are you still experiencing those irritations over small issues, anger, those pangs of jealousy, egos, those phases of depressions and stresses beyond tolerance limits? How do you feel about these changes? Good or bad?

If you find no change in your overall profile or find these changes to be bad and find yourself to be in conditions worse than before, do not hesitate to drop an abusive, expletives ridden, hate mail to me. The least that I can do, is to make a promise that I will not write any more of DIY guides or self-improvement books.

If you are happy about some changes in your lifestyle, your persona, your health and happiness levels or anything else—these may or may not be related to your Yoga learnings, practising and adoption of Yogic way of life—kindly do two things, First, tell others; do your duty to help others in bringing some positive changes in their lives. And second, drop me a mail, describing whatsoever you want to convey.

Thank you for being with me on this beautiful journey. I thoroughly enjoyed your company.

Respectful Regards,

Rakesh Saini

rakeshsaini27@yahoo.com
rakeshsainirathore@gmail.com
@rakeshsaini27